Praise for *Breathing for Warriors*

"*Breathing for Warriors* is the single best resource for the greatest revolution in wellness, performance, and health in our times! Where was this book when I was a young infantry officer trying to max the PT test?"

—Lt. Col. Dave Grossman, author of *On Killing, On Combat,* and *Assassination Generation*

"One of the greatest promises of sport is achieving your highest potential. The best coaches on the planet know this and take lessons learned in high-performance environments and distill them down into essential behaviors for the rest of us mortals. Formula 1–type human performance is more than just entertainment, it is our living laboratory. You are holding the lab notes. Go and see what's possible."

—Dr. Kelly Starrett, DPT, *New York Times* bestselling author and cofounder of The Ready State

"Dr. Belisa is able to explain breathing for athletes with the importance it deserves. Whether you are a pro, amateur, just work out or compete, she is your go-to when it comes to breathing for strength and endurance."

—Juliana Malacarne, bodybuilder and four-time winner of Olympia Women's Physique Showdown

"Dr. Belisa's knowledge of breathing is awesome. I appreciate her ability to translate complex pulmonary information and make it interesting and practical. It is an essential part of physical, emotional, and mental health."

—Laird Hamilton, American big wave surfer

"This book is a wake-up call. Most health problems are caused by what you least expect. If you want to feel better and move with less pain and more power, this is a practical guide that gives readers the ability to do just that."

—Adam Bornstein, *New York Times* bestselling author, chief of nutrition at Ladder, former editorial director at LIVESTRONG, and fitness editor at *Men's Health*

"Rhythmic breathing revitalized my running career and helped me discover my true potential. Whether you're a runner, lifter, or athlete in any other sport, the techniques in *Breathing for Warriors* can help you discover yours."

—Budd Coates, author of *Running on Air,* longtime coach and advisor to *Runner's World* magazine, and four-time Olympic Marathon Trials qualifier

"Replacing reps and time with breaths has been the single biggest game-changer in over a decade for the mobility routines I coach. Discover how much better you'll move and feel when you breathe more efficiently. This book shows you the way."

—Joe DeFranco, world-renowned strength and conditioning coach to NFL, MLB, and NBA players, WWE superstars, UFC fighters, and Olympic and Division I athletes

"Proper breathing is a key part of creating tension, which is the key to strength training. Breathing correctly may seem simple and natural to do, but it's hard to explain. Sabin and Vranich went to great lengths to find the right cues, from the right people, to help you move, lift, and perform better."

——Dan John, lifting and throwing coach, Highland Games competitor and author of *Never Let Go* and several other bestselling books on weight lifting and health

"Breathing is a hot buzzword nowadays, and with that comes a lot of misinformation on the topic. In this book, Vranich and Sabin do a great job of talking about how impactful proper breathing is, and give you actionable and practical advice to implement properly into your own training."

—Mike Robertson, high-performance coach and co-owner of Indianapolis Fitness and Sports Training (I-FAST), named one of America's Top 10 Gyms by *Men's Health*

"*Breathing for Warriors* is not only a 'how-to' but a 'you can' in a world of complex scientific research on the impact of breathing and proper mechanics. Dr. Belisa and Brian have expertly crafted *the* reference guide for breath and its vital importance for all coaches and athletes. This should be everyone's first book when diving into the world of health and fitness literature."

—Sharon A. Moskowitz, Strength and Conditioning Coordinator, USA Wheelchair Rugby

Also by Dr. Belisa Vranich

Breathe: The Simple, Revolutionary 14-Day Program to Improve Your Mental and Physical Health

BREATHING FOR WARRIORS

Master Your Breath to Unlock More Strength, Greater Endurance, Sharper Precision, Faster Recovery, and an Unshakable Inner Game

Dr. Belisa Vranich and Brian Sabin

ST. MARTIN'S
ESSENTIALS

NEW YORK

This book is dedicated to the memory of Shawn Perine, Editor-in-Chief of *Men's Fitness, Muscle & Fitness, Flex,* and *Muscle & Fitness Hers* magazines. Your contribution to the world of fitness and your kindness and generosity as a friend are missed.

The information in this book is not intended to replace the advice of the reader's own physician or other medical professional. You should consult a medical professional in matters relating to health, especially if you have existing medical conditions, and before starting, stopping, or changing the dose of any medication you are taking. Individual readers are solely responsible for their own health-care decisions. The author and the publisher do not accept responsibility for any adverse effects individuals may claim to experience, whether directly or indirectly, from the information contained in this book.

First published in the United States by St. Martin's Essentials, an imprint of St. Martin's Publishing Group

BREATHING FOR WARRIORS. Copyright © 2020 by Dr. Belisa Vranich and Brian Sabin. All rights reserved. Printed in the United States of America. For information, address St. Martin's Publishing Group, 120 Broadway, New York, NY 10271.

www.stmartins.com

Text and graphic design: Casey Altman Design Inc.
Illustrations and notes on illustrations: *The Anatomy of Breathing* by Blandine Calais
Photography: Adam Southard

The Library of Congress Cataloging-in-Publication Data is available upon request.

ISBN 978-1-250-30822-1 (trade paperback)
ISBN 978-1-250-30823-8 (ebook)

Our books may be purchased in bulk for promotional, educational, or business use. Please contact your local bookseller or the Macmillan Corporate and Premium Sales Department at 1-800-221-7945, extension 5442, or by email at MacmillanSpecialMarkets@macmillan.com.

First Edition: March 2020

10 9 8 7

CONTENTS

A NOTE OF CAUTION TO THE READER

This book does not claim to teach medical diagnoses or treatments.

Guidelines and treatment strategies are meant to acquaint you with procedures currently available and the manner in which they may be executed. There are numerous individual differences and unknown conditions in persons with breathing disorders and there are regional variations in the rules which govern the practice of therapy. Therefore, I cannot endorse or take responsibility for any diagnosis or treatment you may make on the basis of the guidelines in this book.

The captions for the illustrations with text from *The Anatomy of Breathing* by Blandine Calais are on page 249.

ACKNOWLEDGMENTS

This book is only as good as its components. It is by no means exhaustive, but it hopes to be the starting point for a very important conversation about the intersection of the mechanics, biochemistry, and psychology of breathing in the world of fitness and well-being. Above all, the underlying framework is collaborative, as the fields of medicine, wellness, and fitness should be. As with the human body, we are only as good as the sum of the parts.

The passion and generosity of the fitness icons and researchers cited is inspiring. I hope that I have done them justice and that this book spurs others to write theirs in turn and add to the field, whether it be breathing science, respiratory physiology, or breathwork.

Daniela Rapp, Cassidy Graham, Lisa Davis, and John Karle of St. Martin's Press, and Peter McGuigan, Kelly Karczuski, Richie Kern, Michael Nardullo, and Sara DeNobrega of Foundry Literary + Media—thank you for believing in this book. I am truly blessed to be able to work with you. Sean Hyson: your feedback and wit are never lost on me. Jason and Jen Ferruggia: I'm so lucky to have you as my LA family and support. Marcus Kowal and Mishel Eder: you have been with me since the very, very beginning; I will be forever grateful for your support. Scott Mann: thank you for sharing your mission, family, and friends with me. Tina Angelotti: thank you for giving me my love of lifting heavy things. Your modeling and feedback on this project were truly appreciated. Steve Kardian: neither this book nor the one before it would ever have made it past a "good idea" to paper without you. Jarard Pearce: you've inspired me with your resilience and by single-handedly becoming a beacon of the breath in New Zealand. Crystal Hernandez of Breathe Beautifully: you've taken what I teach and run with it—you are inspirational. Michael Moschel: your friendship, passion for Tetrahedron Biomechanics, and dedication to your clients will never be forgotten. Stephanie Marango: your friendship and ability to give me perspective are priceless. Jill Miller, my anatomical poet, thank you for lending an ear, a shoulder, and your friendship. Thank you, Desiree Gruber, for truly understanding and believing in the power of the breath. Dr. Ralph and Eugenia Potkin: I could not love you more than I do; your support and encouragement are so appreciated. Jen and Hank Widerstrom: you both were essential parts of this journey; thank you for coming along. My road dog and friend Alyson Khan: thank you for your steadfast friendship. The list of my stalwarts could go on and on, but it would be incomplete if I didn't mention, albeit briefly: Henry Akins, Anthony Lyon, Serena Lee, Gerald Echevarria, Monica Jaggi, Will Giovacchini, Caitlin Mitchell, and Jimmy Lopez. Needless to say, though I shall anyway, this book would never have been possible without the tireless and detailed work of Casey Altman Design Inc.

—*Dr. Belisa Vranich*

should probably thank the asthma I developed in high school for igniting my interest in respiration. We didn't start off on the right foot, breathing and I, but we've grown to understand each other much better over the years.

I definitely owe a debt of gratitude to the sport of running, which showed me that sometimes you can work your way around seemingly insurmountable obstacles—or longtime diagnoses. I'm even more fortunate to have trained under the guidance of Budd Coates, four-time Olympic Marathon Trials qualifier and author of *Running on Air*, whose rhythmic breathing methods showed me just how powerful mindful breathing techniques can be for performance.

But enough yammering on about me. I absolutely must express my gratitude to Belisa for believing in me and bringing me in as a partner on this book. I'd also like to thank Peter McGuigan and the team at Foundry Media for everything they did to bring this work to life.

I feel deeply indebted to all of the trainers, athletes, coaches, and researchers who responded to my many messages and questions with thoughtful responses, including Mike Boyle, Jesse Burdick, Jay Consalvi, Gray Cook, Eric Cressey, Jack Daniels, Joe DeFranco, Tony Gentilcore, Dr. Deborah Graham, Lt. Col. Dave Grossman, Mike Israetel, Joel Jamieson, Deena Kastor, Dr. Sara Lazar, Dr. Daniel Lieberman, Dr. Mitch Lomax, Mary Massery, Sharon A. Moskowitz, C. J. Murphy, Tom Myers, Pia Nilsson, Mark Rippetoe, Dr. Joel Seedman, Louie Simmons and Dave Groves at Westside Barbell, Margaret Smith, Jim "Smitty" Smith, and Pavel Tsatsouline.

I'd like to send an extra-special thank-you to Dr. Jerome Dempsey, Mike Robertson, Dan John, Wim Hof, Ron Hruska, Mike T. Nelson, Jill Miller, Sue Falsone, Alyson Cook, and Brian Mackenzie for being especially generous with their knowledge and time.

I also owe a debt of gratitude to U.S. Navy SEALs Cmdr. (ret.) Mark Divine, whose Box Breathing technique was a life-changer for me. I'd also like to thank Mark W. Muesse for providing me with a gateway to deeper meditative practices.

Thank you to Cristina Goyanes, Amanda Junker Jedeikin, and Sonia Jones at Sonima for providing me with an outlet to explore stories that helped lead to this book. And thank you to Pete Egoscue and Brian Bradley for so many fascinating and fun conversations.

I am deeply thankful to my business partners, Adam and Jordan Bornstein, for all of the support and encouragement they provided me throughout this project. Thank you also to Richelle DeVoe for helping make Pen Name Consulting the incredible family that it is.

Most of all I must thank my wife, Natalie, and our daughters, Piper and Reese. All of you endured far too many weekends without Daddy as I holed up in various coffee shops and libraries to get this project done. I love you all so much. Thank you all for being my rock and my strength, my breath and my life.

Lastly, I'd like to thank you for reading this.

—*Brian Sabin*

INTRODUCTION

This is the book that will change everything. *Breathing for Warriors* is not a feel-good inspirational book, and although breathing can be magical, beautiful, and otherworldly, this book is not about any of that. *Breathing for Warriors* explains *a system* and gives warriors—athletes, first responders—the outline and instructions for how to breathe in a mechanically optimal way for the unique demands of their sport or line of duty. And after you learn the whys and hows and are moving in a structurally sound way, you will learn how to strengthen your breathing muscles. The results will not only be increased endurance, strength, and precision, but also better support of the nervous system—even of your emotional well-being, from the bottom up.

Everything we learn is built on the shoulders of others, and this system is built on those belonging to experts on ventilation, respiration, and breathwork—from different points in history and diverse vantage points. Our references are by no means exhaustive; rather, they are the starting point of a new paradigm where we consider the breath in sports and performance and, hopefully, add to new science and theory. Breathing can be divided into three camps: Breath-Induced Trance Meditation (e.g., holotropic breathwork), Respiration (at the cellular level related to CO_2), and Mechanical Ventilation. What we look at in this book, then, are the mechanics, muscles, and posture of breathing (ventilation).

The following is a series of principles on which this book is based, inspired by the seven principles that Russian Special Operations Chief Instructor Vladimir Vasiliev expounds in his book, *Let*

Every Breath . . . Secrets of the Russian Breath Masters. As does Vasiliev, I believe that these principles apply to "every waking moment of your life," in addition to how warriors should breathe while working out or while recovering.

1. *The Principle of Anatomical Congruence.* The goal is that your breathing be biomechanically sound (anatomically congruent). To do this, you consider your Location of Movement (LOM) and Range of Motion (ROM). LOM should be at the middle of the body where the diaphragm is located and the lungs are the biggest. ROM measures abdominothoracic respiratory flexibility—what in medical literature has been called "thoracic excursion." Together the LOM and ROM give you your Breathing IQ or B-IQ.

2. *The Principle of Breathing IQ.* Having a *functional* grading system for the mechanics of your breathing (anatomical congruence) makes improvement possible and practical. A summary of medical literature shows that using *primary* breathing muscles (diaphragm, intercostals, and abs/obliques) impacts your entire well-being, including pain management, blood pressure, digestive and back health, performance, and longevity.

3. *The Principle of Movement Integrity.* Breathing is the most basic movement we make. All other movement builds on breathing, owing to the fact that it is the foundation for any other complex movement pattern. When breathing is anatomically congruous, movements (whether they be in dance or when picking up a pencil) have integrity. Locomotive pairing—supple and stable movement—is predicated on harnessing the breath.

4. *The Principle of Psychology and Breathing.* There is a psychological element to inhales and exhales. Breathing and emotions are *bidirectional* (your mood affects your breathing and your breathing affects your mood). Becoming aware of the psychosocial factors that have affected your breathing is a part of influencing change. These include:

a. Our body's translation of the environment, especially given technology and chronic stress (posture and bracing)

b. Negative feelings about one's body (height or weight)

c. Myths and misunderstandings about the respiratory system

d. Life experiences where you resorted to fight, flight, or freeze

5. *The Principle of an Amnestic Diaphragm.* Bracing—and bracing well—can keep your back safe when you lift. But bracing as an all-day, everyday posture is deleterious to your physical *and* mental health. Bracing, guarding, "sucking it in"—*emotional corsets, muscular corsets*—all affect the proper mechanics of the breath. Unfortunately, the result is an inhibited diaphragm that is locked up or *amnestic.* It gives the body no choice but to breathe vertically, or apically, using auxiliary neck and shoulder muscles. The symptoms are so far from the source—breathing—that we don't recognize them as being rooted in the breakdown of the middle part of "the machine."

6. *The Principle of Perfect Trifecta.* The pelvic floor, thoracic diaphragm, and connection by the psoas muscles create the framework of biomechanically sound breathing. These muscles frame the digestive, spinal, and urogenital systems. A breath supports healthy organs, better center of balance, and healthier spine and gut. Reversing dysfunctional mechanics in order to give the diaphragm its throne back as a primary breathing muscle has mind-blowing health and performance consequences. The diaphragm supports the lungs and the heart from below, and the lower back, digestive organs, and pelvic floor from above. This change of health habit is like no other since it's self-reinforcing—you used to breathe this way, and your body wants to breathe this way.

7. *The Principle of Detoxification.* While the liver and the kidneys are the body's major detoxifying organs, the diaphragm is

the body's main detoxifying muscle. Its widening and narrowing of the middle of the body enhances circulation, digestion, and the movement of lymph.

8. *The Popeye Principle.* Popeye's barrel chest doesn't show strength, it shows high residual air. As a person ages, the efficiency and strength of the exhale, the narrowing of body and rib cage, is critical. Otherwise, ossification occurs and the exhale suffers, meaning the person retains more residual air and experiences *air hunger,* one of the most misunderstood and undertreated symptoms in doctors' offices and hospitals today.

9. *The Principle of Pedagogical Breath Retraining.* Taking a belly breath is the first step in understanding and learning circumferential Diaphragmatic Breathing (measured by abdominothoracic respiratory flexibility). Successful dismantling of bad breathing habits (e.g., bracing) and relearning better mechanics require multisensory, pedagogically sound instruction. Otherwise, the instructions to "take a deep breath" are so laden with myth and misunderstanding that they are ineffective or result in only short-term change. Owing to its teaching and kinesthetic component, this principle elicits an immediate sense of calm.

10. *The Principle of Efficiency.* A mechanically sound diaphragmatic (horizontal) breath is more efficient owing to the fact that more air passes in and out of the body in one breath than with an apical or Vertical Breath. Breath patterns and pace will become more natural, and a balance of the breath is more possible when the body is breathing in an anatomically congruous way.

11. *The Principle of Ten Pounds.* The combined weight of the correct principal breathing muscles is over ten pounds. *Your biggest enemy is perceived fatigue, which often comes from undertrained breathing muscles.* Sports science has clearly found that breathing-muscle training delays fatigue. Stronger breathing muscles mean more "fuel," better endurance and conditioning (separate from cardio, which works out the heart).

12. *The Principle of Active Recovery.* Regeneration, adaptation, and

peak performance can only be achieved if active recovery is included in training. Breathing exercises and meditation are integral parts of recovery.

13. *The Principle of Arousal Control.* Breathing is the mind/body connection. It can be cathartic, activating, or calming. From where you breathe holds the key to controlling the nervous system and stress. Treating stress and mental health effectively includes addressing the breath.

14. *The Principle of "The Machine."* Take care of the machine and the machine will take care of you. Make sure your head and hips are where they should be, and that the middle of your body is flexible. Activated, strong breathing muscles enable you to inhale and exhale better; in addition, they keep you upright, balanced, and less prone to injury.

> *Our mission is to integrate breathing biomechanics and breathing-muscle strength into clinical assessment protocols and performance regimens.*

Disrupted breathing biomechanics is a public health problem like smoking, sedentarism, obesity, stress, and mental health issues. Addressing and fixing the biomechanics of breathing—rather than "rearranging the deck chairs on the *Titanic*"[1]—can alleviate pain and the effects of stress for what research biochemist-turned-author Robb Wolf calls the tsunami of neurodegenerative disorders, such as MS and Parkinson's.[2] Adding the B-IQ (LOM/ROM) to health assessments with standardized exercises to repair it can have a deep impact on the cost, quality, and outcome of care.

By following these principles and the practical exercises, at the end of this book you should be able to say *yes* to the following:

- Are you breathing in a way that is biomechanically sound, anatomically congruous?

---

1   Quote attributed to Joseph Eger, "Listening to the Vibes," *The New York Times*, May 15, 1972.

2   Personal correspondence, June 5, 2018.

- Are you breathing in a way that simultaneously energizes and detoxifies you?
- Are you breathing in a way that gives you choices as far as your state of arousal? Not just the ends of the sympathetic or parasympathetic spectrum (your state of arousal from calm to panicked), but the combinations in between that vary in terms of alertness and vigilance or calmness?
- Are you breathing in a way that supports your mental game, your ability to access flow, your ability to recover and regenerate from day to day?
- Are you breathing in a way that gives you stability, that gives your movement integrity, and that keeps you injury-free?

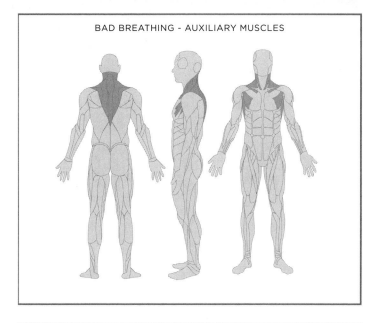

BAD BREATHING - AUXILIARY MUSCLES

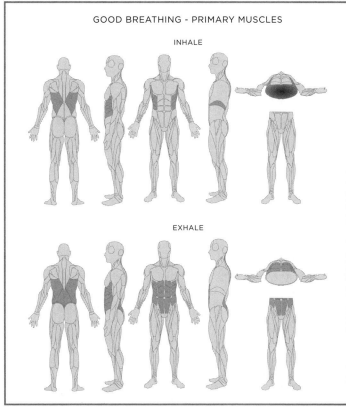

GOOD BREATHING - PRIMARY MUSCLES

INHALE

EXHALE

3

---

3   Bristling at the idea of "bad" vs. "good" breathing? Relax. You need different ways to breathe depending on the situation, but the point is that your primary breathing muscles should be your main breathing muscles.

1

BREATHING FIRE: A NEW PARADIGM FOR BETTER PERFORMANCE

Fatigue is your worst enemy as an athlete—pro or amateur. It's not lack of heart motivation or "not wanting it bad enough." It's a question of running out of energy, of not being able to catch your breath. You don't pay attention to your breathing when you are just walking around; however, you have no choice but to notice it when things go wrong. You've been there. You're in the thick of things and you're breathing as hard as you can, and it feels as if you just can't get enough air. Then doubt creeps in. You try to shake it off, but soon you cross that line from no longer playing to win to just praying to make it through with your dignity intact. "Fatigue makes cowards of us all" are words attributed to both Gen. George Patton and legendary NFL coach Vince Lombardi. Both knew that when you're tired and can't catch your breath, you are done, no matter how talented you are, how desperately you want to win, or how well you've trained for that moment.

While most people turn to cardio, the answer to running out of energy is strengthening your breathing muscles. Here, you will learn how to train those breathing muscles so that you'll be able to tap into energy reserves you didn't know you had.

PERCEIVED FATIGUE

Scientific studies have shown that respiratory muscle training has indubitably led to better performance. Often, the heavy, can't-catch-your-breath tired feeling has to do with the very breathing muscles fatiguing. "Perceived fatigue" is the sensation of being tired, but one that is fleeting; often, it leaves you angry as you look back and see you just needed a few seconds to recover.

You may ask if breathing was, well, "just breathing," wouldn't you be able to do breathing exercises indefinitely? As you'll see later, you can't. The breathing muscle exercises we'll do will make you sweat and cramp, and you will feel exhausted (your muscles have been overloaded, as needed for growth). The result: an almost immediate change in your endurance when you run, swim, or just recover between sets.

> "Most people find the whole area of breathing completely mystifying and have no notion of how breathing is brought about, how it responds to exercise, how and why these responses differ at different exercise intensities, or how the lungs themselves respond to training."
>
> — Alison McConnell, author of *Breathe Strong, Perform Better*

WAIT. BREATHING MUSCLES?

You have about ten pounds of breathing muscles just languishing; that is to say, not being trained functionally. You are not training these muscles when you do cardio. Your lungs are burning on that obstacle course, but are you "training" them? Nope. The notion that you are working your breathing muscles when training couldn't be further from the truth. Why? To work out a muscle you have to push it to exhaustion, and to do this you have to train breathing muscles separately from your sport. If you don't work on your inspiratory and expiratory breathing muscles separately, you are running on three cylinders. By overlooking breathing, you are unknowingly sleeping on a mattress full of money.

The spongy, angel cake–like tissues of your lungs are just that—a veiny, leaf-like network of airways within them. But few people pay attention to the steaming pistons and engines that bring air to the tiny pink air sacs (the alveoli) where the exchange of oxygen and carbon dioxide takes place. The network of alveoli is beautiful, complex, and delicate architecture; however, it isn't something that powers itself. On their own, the lungs do nothing. They are motionless slabs of oblong-shaped sponge, but they are surrounded by a fortress-like infrastructure of muscles. There is an entire powerful muscular mechanism working behind every inhale and exhale.

When your breathing muscles are strong, you can breathe easier and exercise longer at harder levels of effort, and the experience feels easier. The burn or heaviness in your arms and legs will happen later in the game. You even bounce back faster from tough, all-out efforts. Neglecting these muscles is like going to the gym, passing by all the weights, and spending the whole time doing forearm curls.

We've summarized the research, the history, and the most common problems. We've interviewed the top experts in the field, special operations people, martial artists, sports celebrities, and trainers from around the world. We've translated stodgy academic articles into practical advice. We're going to talk about gladiators, why it's better to be savage, the dumb things you are doing, and smart things that you are not.

DO THIS NOW

Imagine 600 big water cooler bottles lined up. All in all, you're talking about your breathing muscles working to move 3,000 gallons of air (or 11,000 liters) in and out of your body every day.

Be an experimenter. Breathing training delays fatigue throughout the body, keeping the working muscles in the arms and legs from feeling heavy and burning. Before you start the training, we recommend picking a marker of your endurance: running time, a rowing distance, or a consistent "hit the wall" time.

EXERCISE SCIENCE: WHAT TOOK THE WORLD SO LONG?

If you hadn't given much thought to your breathing before opening the pages of *Breathing for Warriors*, that's not your fault. Exercise science is just catching up with the research studies that look at breathing and its potential in sports and fitness. Current manuals from the certification organizations that oversee modern strength and conditioning rarely discuss breathing in depth; most jam any discussion about breathing and respiration into a section on cardiovascular development with a shout-out to heart rate, and leave it at that. The omission can be chalked up to a combination of myths and misunderstandings, the biggest one of which is that breathing can't be trained. At least that was the line of thinking until about twenty years ago, when troves of studies began to show that breathing effort is unequivocally a limiting factor in exercise, and that when you strengthen breathing muscles, that effort decreases (and therefore your limits expand).

The *Journal of Sports Science & Medicine*, the *European Journal of Applied Psychology*, and the *British Journal of Sports Medicine* are a few of the academic journals that have documented how training breathing muscles betters performance. Athletic breathing experts—such as Alison Mc-Connell and Mitch Lomax—have worked with hundreds of cyclists, swimmers, runners, and climbers, publishing articles such as "Adaptation of Endurance Training with a Reduced Breathing Frequency" and "Inspiratory muscle training, altitude, and arterial oxygen desaturation: A preliminary investigation." Breathing training helps you boost your endurance *and* helps you recover from sprints and high-altitude hikes.

> "The diaphragm is the pneumatic hub of your body. Its health impacts every system on a macro/micro level. It has unseen contributions to posture, performance, gait, emotional regulation, digestion, elimination, circulation, immunity, and respiration. It's directly connected to ever-popular trunk muscles that are a training target in the #fitness world. The muscle building (bigger is better) bias can leave the diaphragm without balanced mobility to its neighbors."
>
> — Jill Miller, anatomy expert and creator of Yoga Tune Up[1]

WHY IS IT TAKING SO LONG FOR THIS TO BE COMMON KNOWLEDGE?

1. First of all, the vocabulary used to discuss breathing training targeted at the general public has been romantic, vague, or woo-woo, so most people tuned out. Additionally, much of the discussion about breathing training has been reserved for breathing disorders like COPD or asthma.

2. It takes almost a decade for information to go from study results to classrooms to playing fields. You have probably just started to hear about breathing training over the last year. If you look at the dates for some of the formative studies, we are right on target. You are going to be hearing a lot about

---

1   Interview, May 18, 2018.

breathing, respiration, and ventilation in the performance arena over the next decade.

3. The effects of living in the era of information technology and the sudden ("sudden" when compared to the entire history of mankind) change in the body's posture and stress brought about by constant information are both acute and insipid.

4. Many medical presenters have quoted the two-generational Framingham study involving an enormous cohort. From it, we have learned priceless information about cardiac health, vascular health, and lifestyle dangers. But while it touted that breathing was an important factor in health and longevity, no one gave us any practical cues or straightforward instructions. The myths around breathing are numerous.

THREE MYTHS ABOUT BREATHING AND EXERCISE PERFORMANCE

For years sports scientists incorrectly believed that breathing did not limit physical performance. Recent research has proven this to be incorrect.

MYTH: Breathing muscles are highly evolved and do not exhibit fatigue.

TRUTH: Breathing muscles tire just like any other muscle in your body, and if they are not trained, they will contribute to whether or not your endurance and conditioning is peak (you just don't feel the "burn" like you do with other muscles).

MYTH: Oxygen delivery is the limiting factor in performance.

TRUTH: The limiting factor is your ability to sustain intensity while resisting fatigue and to tolerate the building of lactate produced during high-intensity work.

MYTH: You can't increase lung size, lung volume, or enhance the ability to transfer oxygen to the blood.

TRUTH: By breathing diaphragmatically, you can ensure you are maximizing what you have, rather than breathing vertically, which takes in a significantly smaller amount of air.

WHY NOW?

Mechanics and muscles have received more attention recently because of a convergence of interest in kettlebells, free diving, first responder and veteran health, forest fires, and such feats as Ross Edgley's swimming around England, Julie Gautier's six-minute dance in the world's deepest pool, and Wim Hof's barefoot marathon in the Arctic Circle. Specifically, within the sports world, there's been a growing awareness of how breathing impacts every movement an athlete makes owing to the achievement of pioneers such as Ron Hruska, Tom Myers, Gray Cook, Donna Farhi, Mary Massery, Erik Peper, Katy Bowman, Robert Fried, Blandine Calais, and Leon Chaitow, to name a few.

A NEW PARADIGM IN PERFORMANCE

Welcome to the new frontier in health, fitness, and sports performance. The frontier lies in between pulmonology (the study of the respiratory tract and lungs) and breathwork or conscious breathing, and deals with biomechanics, psychology, and the nervous system.

Attend any sports conference this year and you'll see how peak performance, optimization, movement recovery, resilience, and mental health are the top topics. What is the foundation of all of these? Breathing. The practicality of this is explained in this book.

Training your breathing and your breathing muscles is part of a new paradigm in performance. And this is only the beginning of the

> "Breathing is the only system in the body that is both automatic and also under our control. That is not an accident of nature, not a coincidence—it's an invitation, an opportunity to take part in our own nature and evolution. There are details in the way you breathe that you probably have never observed or explored, and these details are like doorways that can lead to new and profound abilities. The fact is breathwork is a major skill set if you want to become a high-performing individual and enhance every aspect of your life."
>
> — Dan Brulé, author of *Just Breathe*

> ## MEDITATION'S LITTLE BROTHER
>
> For years, "breathwork" has tagged along with meditation or yoga. Traditionally, it had to do with trance-induced breathing (e.g., rebirthing or transformational). At the other extreme are respiratory physiologists who treat such disorders as COPD and emphysema.

conversation. A monumental shift in the world's understanding of the lungs and ventilation, and the muscles that power them, is coming. Over the next few years, as practical guidelines start to integrate what scientific studies have shown, strong breathing will be seen as every bit as important as cardiovascular health. *Breathing for Warriors* will enable you to be an active participant when people talk about the importance of breathing, and you'll also be able to leave with a method to assess and train your clients and athletes—and it will help you improve your own breathing.

And perhaps best of all, the athletes and warriors who train their breathing muscles will move faster, lift heavier, and perform better.

2

CHOOSE YOUR ATHLETIC SUPERPOWER

Around 300 BC, a Greek named Erasistratus of Chios discovered that the lungs did not work on their own, and that they required muscles in order to function. Further, centuries ago people thought the body's arteries were hollow and carried air throughout the body. Then about a century later, Galen, a Roman surgeon and philosopher, documented how arteries were filled with blood, not air. It was through his work with wounded gladiators that Galen (a friend of Emperor Marcus Aurelius, whom you know from Stoic philosophy or the movie *Gladiator*) initiated the study of human respiration that informs the foundation of modern medicine. He would perform public vivisections on animals in order to prove his theories about anatomy. In one experiment, Galen used bellows to inflate the lungs of a dead animal. His work with gladiators and animal corpses alike informed much of the thinking around human respiration.

Much of what's known today in the context of sport and exercise stems from the work of a pioneer and giant in the field of exercise physiology: Englishman Archibald Vivian Hill.[1] He and German biochemist Otto Meyerhof explained the difference between the anaerobic and aerobic systems, and consequently shared a Nobel Prize in Medicine in 1922 for their discovery.

Hill continued working in sports and identified the phenomenon known as Excess Post-exercise Oxygen Consumption or EPOC; that is to say, that your body uses more oxygen than it has and must "catch up" after you stop moving.

Hill's tests often involved running, and at times must have been

---

1   Author of several weighty tomes; e.g., *Muscular Activity; Muscular Movement in Man; Living Machinery; The Ethical Dilemma of Science and Other Writings.*

ALMOST A PINT

Are you close to or over twenty-nine? The average person's lung capacity starts to decline between their late 20s and mid-30s, and decreases by about 380 milliliters for men and slightly less for women every decade. That's like losing a three-quarters-full pint glass of air (or even more). The biggest reason you've never thought about this is that you can't feel your diaphragm burn like a repped-out quad. It's a completely different type of muscle that doesn't render the fatigue feedback you are used to. Your entire point of reference for muscle building is useless here.

uncomfortable for the participants. For example, in order to determine how much oxygen a runner required in order to hit a certain speed, he asked a fleet-footed study participant (the guy could run the 100-meter dash in 10.6 seconds) to run distances up to 120 meters while holding his breath. Then immediately after crossing the line, he'd lie down and breathe into a bag. Hill could then measure exactly how much oxygen the runner had needed to cover the distance he did at the speed he'd hit.

A late '90s/early 2000s series of studies investigated respiratory muscle fatigue and how it affects locomotor muscles.[2] It was at this same time that a new host of pressures—from technological to psychological—changed the human body in ways that actively make breathing more challenging. We'll talk about that in the next chapter. For now, let's look at you.

NOW YOU COME INTO THE PICTURE—THE PLAN

So here is what we are going to do: get a baseline measurement on you, finesse the mechanics (make sure you are using the right muscles), then strengthen those right muscles. If you want to do the math to get a grade, go for it. Want to have a general sense of things? We'll give you info to do that.

This is all practical and science-based, so make sure you log your baseline numbers, whether they be when you hit a wall when doing an endurance sport, how fast you recover, the stability of a lift, your mental health (anxiety), or ability to recover between training, so that you can see how this changes as you train your breathing muscles.

---

2   For example, studies by Lee Romer et al. in the *Journal of Physiology*; in the *Journal of Sports Sciences*; and in *Medicine & Science in Sports & Exercise*.

HOW DO YOU WANT TO IMPROVE YOUR PERFORMANCE?

This book isn't the one to read while curled up in your pajamas sipping hot cocoa. It's a practical system where you need to be involved and assertive. So, start by taking a big fat Sharpie or high-lighter and circle the options below that apply to you. (Whoever reads this book after you can deal with it.)

☐ *Endurance*: I want to be able to run longer, faster. I want to be able to spar and have a steadier stream of energy so "run-ning out of gas" is not something I am anxious about. I want to feel as if I have reserves that I can always tap into, so that when I need to "dig deep," I can.

I want to _____

_____

_____

☐ *Strength*: I want to lift and feel as if I'm working off a super strong base, so I can consider adding more weight. I want to feel as if my breath is helping the movement and making it feel integrated. I want to feel as if my stability is rock solid and protecting me from injury. I want to have a better sense of when I can do another rep, or when it's ego and I need to back off. I want to be able to recover between sets and feel fresh for the next one.

I want to _____

_____

_____

☐ *Precision*: I want to be able to be more consistent in my game (whether it's golf, archery, shooting, or pool), so that my per-formance is not about the weather, my equipment, or my mood. I want to be able to switch off the mental chatter and focus regardless of the distractions around me. I want to be able to keep my focus consistent, stop mulling about my last shot, and focus entirely on the present one.

I want to _____

_____

_____

☐ *Recovery*: I want to be able to recover between sets. I want to be able to recover day to day, so I'm less exhausted tomorrow because of my hard workout today. I want my recovery time between circuits to be less. I want the number of breaths I take to reboot to be less, so I am ready to go again faster. I want to feel as if I really recover and regenerate between workouts, not just rest. I want to be able to lower my heart rate and catch my breath faster. I want to feel fresh the next day, not dragging.

I want to _____

_____

_____

By the way, "all of the above" is an acceptable answer.

GET A MEASURE

Treat this like a number on the scale: your personal best squat, your daily 5K time, your heart rate. Note the exact moment you start to get winded on a rower, or your handicap in golf. By the end, you'll discover what hundreds of other "tip of the spear" athletes who've ventured out to try breathing training already know: proper breathing is an athletic superpower, and strong breathing muscles supercharge it.

WHAT'S NEXT? MECHANICS. THEN STRENGTH.
GET IT RIGHT. THEN MAKE IT STRONG.

After you've laid the foundation of the right mechanics of proper breathing, you'll put your new skills to work in the following sections.

- *Breathing for Endurance (chapters 8, 9, and 10):* Supercharge your conditioning significantly and quickly—without adding cardio. If you have to manage your energy over an extended amount of time, or you are a runner, cyclist, swimmer, or athlete where there is no pacing but you have to accelerate and decelerate quickly, you will definitely want to spend some time here. We'll talk about everything from pacing to energy systems. Get a baseline as a measure of endurance, be it how many laps you can swim, your usual gassing point on a run, etc. Make sure your mechanics are good (that is, make sure your location of movement and range of motion that make up the Breathing IQ is good), then time yourself or count reps, and just as with any exercise, add difficulty and track it. Slam through these exercises with the intensity of any other type of workout. Don't just observe. Write down and track the changes in the level of effort, times, or distance.

> ### HOW DO THE PROS DO IT?
>
> The elite of the elite performers always integrate the breath. Some do it consciously, and to some it comes easily, unconsciously. Whether it's a speech or a kettlebell sequence, watch someone do a movement pattern that is seamless. Most pros will explain the "feeling" and talk in terms of "flow," but they can't explain the "how." We will.

- *Breathing for Strength (chapters 11, 12, and 13):* Breathing horizontally means increased stability and power (and therefore less risk of injury). We'll summarize the most common mistakes with breathing and strength training, and the best bracing techniques. We've interviewed top athletes in the field and included their experience and recommendations when it comes to breathing. We'll review "locomotor joining" (the direction of breath for the top gym movements). We'll address recovering between sets for more energy. For recovery between days, make sure you head to that chapter too.

- *Breathing for Precision (chapters 14 and 15):* Whether it's a bull's-eye or a stellar short game, we'll give you practical advice and exercises in order to teach you to recognize when you are the stillest and can be most accurate. This chapter will give you practical exercises in order to consistently find your "natural pause"—whether you are a bowhunter or a billiards player, and will show you how to discover how to tune into a higher level when every millimeter matters.

- *Breathing for Recovery (chapter 16):* The newest research in the field is focusing on recovery and regeneration. The easiest and most effective recovery is reached by adding a short active meditation to your day. This means, long term, better detoxification of your body, which lets you heal faster so that you can go hard again.

- *Between Your Ears (chapter 17):* The last section covers mental health, inner game, resilience, and public speaking. If you are injured, hard-breathing exercises can help you heal faster, maintain your conditioning, and protect you from depression. Breathing is the connection between mind and body. Take your confidence up a level, or ten, with proven practices for gaining mastery of nervousness and self-doubt. Mental game has always been the most elusive factor in sports, which is why there are so many books, opinions, and experts in the field. But if you get to the very core of the connection between your mind and your body, you have your breathing. Your ability to flow—on demand—is intimately connected to how you breathe.

You will discover that each chapter offers you the fundamental techniques and exercises you can use to make your breathing

---

> **MOVE STEALTHILY**
>
> Poor breathing patterns have been linked to poor performance in other activities. For example, a 2014 study found that people who displayed signs of a breathing pattern disorder were also likely to score poorly on the Functional Movement Screen (FMS).[3]

---

3 FMS is a system developed by Gray Cook, MSPT, OCS, CSCS, an eloquent and passionate expert on breathing and how it relates to movement.

complement or support your sport or activity across the different athletic modalities. *Breathing for Warriors*, then, will start by:

- Teaching you how to give yourself a functional test for breathing.
- Teaching you how to use the right muscles when you breathe.
- Training the muscles.
- Tracking the results. Watch your goal time or "personal best" improve.

3

HOW MODERN LIVING TOOK OUR BREATH AWAY

BREATHE LIKE A SAVAGE

In an article in *Scientific American*, Robin Lloyd points out that "Exactly what causes dysfunctional breathlessness is uncertain, but many experts suspect that it originates from biomechanical or psychological disturbances, or some combination of the two. One possible culprit is breathing that stems from the upper chest rather than the entire chest and abdomen."[1]

Just last year *Science News* published a virtual 3-D construction of a Neanderthal rib cage, revealing that early man had a *larger* diaphragm, *more* lung capacity, and *greater* stability than modern man. A separate study carried out in London found that Neanderthal's nasal passages were about 29 percent *larger* than those of modern humans—meaning they were able to move air through their nose at a higher rate, one that could help to sustain "an active lifestyle involving much huffing and puffing." In addition, primitive man had *less* intercostal innervation (which came about later for better control of exhale and hence, formation of sentences) and a longer neck to adapt the voice box.

Modern man, on the other hand, chooses to breathe vertically more often; that is to say, he is an upper chest and shoulder breather. However, apical breathing is not the only nonsensical function that "civilized man" has acquired; it seems he is "the only creature who sleeps with open mouth."[2]

Quite recently in the history of man, breathing went from using primary breathing muscles to

> "We have paid a high price for civilization. The savage, today, breathes naturally, unless he has been contaminated by the habits of civilized man."
>
> — William Walker Atkinson, author of *Science of Breath*

---

1   Lloyd, Robin. "Gasping for Air." *Scientific American* 316 (2017):26–27.

2   Zornitsa Valcheva, et al. "The role of mouth breathing on dentition development and formation"; *The Journal of IMAB*, (2018) Jan.-Mar. 24(1).

using secondary breathing muscles as primary ones. A new host of pressures over the last few decades—from technological to psychological—have changed the human body in ways that actively make breathing more challenging.

What a profound shift in the way we are designed to perform the most important bodily function! Your average inhale consistently relies on auxiliary muscles at the top of the body, rather than Circumferential Abdominothoracic Breathing where the diaphragm and the biggest part of the lungs are. Any anatomy enthusiast would shudder at the possible consequences, the most common of which is a sense of breathlessness, which leaves one feeling as if one can't breathe as fully as one should, or as strongly as one did when younger.

> Have you noticed how psychology keeps making its way into a topic usually dealing with mechanics and anatomy? Breathing has a *psychological* and mechanical aspect to it, apart from the emotional bi-directionality—that your breathing affects your nervous system and emotions and vice versa. Why our breathing has gone "awry" has to do with myths, misunderstandings, and culture.

WHY "TAKE A DEEP BREATH" DOESN'T REALLY RESULT IN ONE

Ringside, what is the word one hears most often? *Breathe!* But what comes to mind when you are told to take a deep breath? Usually, you imagine looking upward, filling

---

3   Interview on April 10, 2019. Goodman is known for his use of thumbs and pinkie hand position as a "measuring stick," while hinging at the hips and elongating (not crunching) the back.

If you think we mammals are the most evolved in terms of breathing, think again. An article in the *European Respiratory Journal* reports that some 300 million years ago, the ancestors of modern reptiles emerged from the sea and were committed to air breathing. The two great classes of vertebrates with high levels of maximal oxygen consumption—the mammals and birds—subsequently evolved. A remarkable feature of these two divergent evolutionary lines is that, although the physiology of many organ systems shows many similarities, the lungs are radically different, with birds being the *more* advanced.

> THE DECOMPRESSIVE QUALITIES OF THE BREATH (OR HOW TO DECOMPRESS IN A COMPRESSED WORLD)
>
> "As a Neanderthal, much of your rib cage was behind you," says Dr. Eric Goodman. "Your lungs can't think on their own, can only follow orders. Your torso is supposed to be expansive and you have to re-educate the rib cage. Levels and pulleys that pull the cage are the generators, they have to contract and relax."[3]

"Breathing profoundly influences the very way that we experience our lives. If we are breathing to merely survive, any method will suffice. Breathing effectively will give you dominion over your states of consciousness. As a martial arts instructor, I have observed the breathing patterns of thousands of students. Children usually breathe diaphragmatically when they are passive and immediately following intense intervals of activity. Adults tend to puff out their chests, for one reason or another, and they appear to be tense during periods of passivity, and have a hard time calming their respiration immediately following demanding physical training. It doesn't self-correct. Diaphragmatic breathing requires practice. When the skill is cultivated, individuals are able to induce moods of their choosing through breathing patterns that are appropriate to the desired result. People who learn to breathe effectively will experience their lives accordingly."[4]

— Thomas Clifford, black belt,
Emperado kajukenbo and
Gracie jiu-jitsu

your upper chest, and raising your shoulders. All wrong. But why do people do this? The first reason is that the collective understanding of what a deep breath looks like is incorrect. The image that comes to mind for a "deep breath" couldn't be further from the truth. To correct this, you have to add some psychology; that is to say, understand/uncover/examine what the confusing cues are and the misunderstandings that made you believe them, then get some facts and rectify the problem.

DETHRONING OF THE DIAPHRAGM: THE SAGA

Take any machine and disconnect a main component from the engine. In the case of a human being, the main component would be the large muscle right underneath the heart and above the entire digestive system—the diaphragm. The ripple of dysfunction would spread from high to low; as a result, the consequences are so far from the source one may not recognize it. Your endurance not being what it used to be, that nagging back pain . . . and you don't complain, but rather just keep disconnecting, numbing out, or justifying it as old age, bad genes, or bad luck.

THE DIAPHRAGM: MISUNDERSTOOD AND MALIGNED

We can't see our lungs, we can't see air, and we can't feel the diaphragm because it doesn't have nerve endings like other muscles. It's been likened to a distasteful toilet plunger, shaped like

---

4   Interview on February 15, 2019.

an unbalanced squid that's hard to draw. To make matters worse, sports references that discuss strength omit the diaphragm—it's a hard one to include in the "muscle man" image, one that only shows "exterior" pecs, glutes, abs, and such. So, this massively important, regal muscle is relegated to the status of an unnecessary add-on, much the way most folks feel about their pinkie toes or appendix. We know it's there, but we are not sure why. When functioning correctly, this King of Muscles, the diaphragm, connects directly to the lower back and affects the health of the spine. Think of it like a massive hand above the digestive system, kneading it much like bread, from above. And if that weren't enough, diaphragmatic breathing also impacts your center of gravity, your ability to detox lactic acid and control your stress—because of its direct connection with the nervous system.

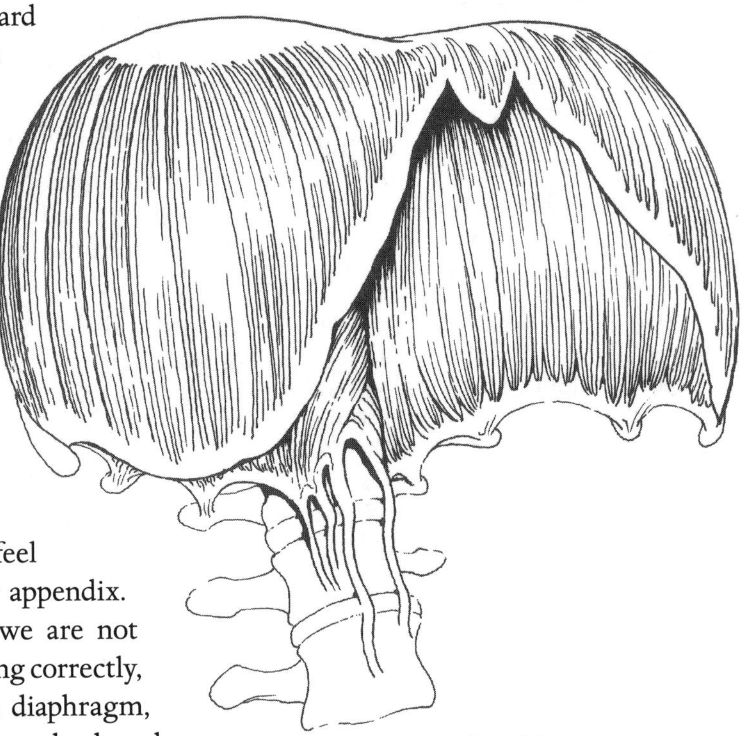

Figure 3.1

Now bear with me, because I have to get very specific as far as our muscles are concerned. The diaphragm, intercostals, transverse abdominis, and obliques are among the primary muscles of breathing. For the inhale, the main muscles of inspiration are the diaphragm and outer intercostals, whereas for the exhale, it's the inner intercostals, obliques, and abs. The sternocleidomastoid, upper trapezius, and upper pecs

Vitalic Breathing by Thomas Robert Gaines was published in 1921, almost 100 years ago. He warned what a constricted "civilized" breath would do. Breathing like a "savage," in a more natural and healthy way, but also with savage intention and desire will, oddly enough, make you a more evolved optimal human. Correct the mechanics, strengthen the muscles, then do what you do best and see your numbers get better.

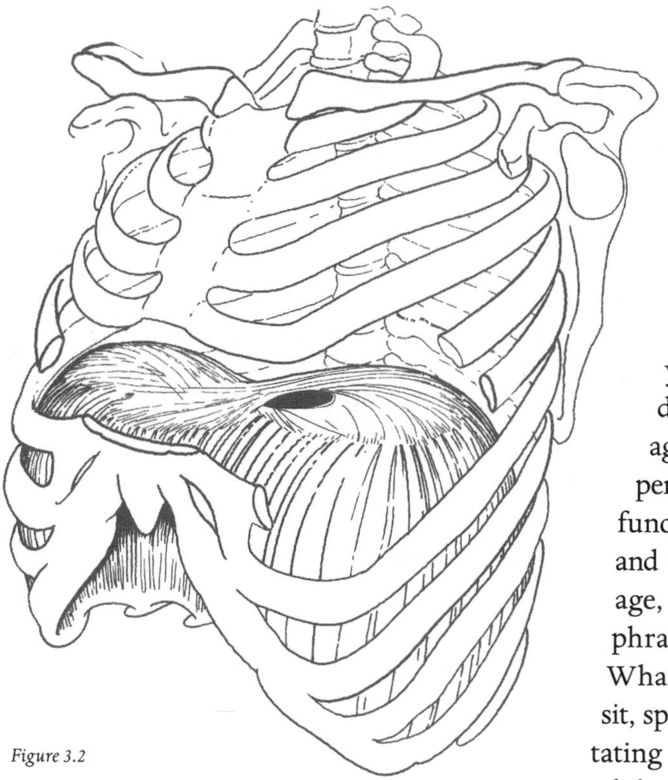

Figure 3.2

are accessory muscles, but modern man is using auxiliary muscles as primary muscles. And this change happens at a very specific age. In a 2017 *Men's Fitness* article on breathing, author and colleague Sean Hyson aptly described how the perfect childhood breath becomes "corrupted."[5] Last year, I conducted a study on 158 children ages 2–11 and found that the age of change from an anatomically perfect breath to a mimicking, dysfunctional one occurs at exactly five and a half years of age. Prior to that age, children breathe using their diaphragm without shame or bracing. What causes the change? Starting to sit, spending less time on the floor, imitating parents and superheroes, stress, and shame about weight/body image—in short, bracing, guarding, and sucking it in. What is your story? What are the myths or experiences that have affected your breathing?

WHAT SHOULD BE HAPPENING AS PER OUR DESIGN?

Do you really understand the mechanics of your breathing muscles? A complex interplay exists during inhalation: The diaphragm flattens and the increased intra-abdominal pressure causes an outward expansion of the abdomen. As the diaphragm continues to move, its attachment to the lower ribs causes the lower ribs to expand horizontally. In other words, the rib cage opens. Make sure you can visualize this in your mind's eye.

---

5   Hyson, Sean. *The Men's Health Encyclopedia of Muscle*. Rodale, 2018.

A dysfunctional breathing pattern exists when there is minimal circumferential (meaning some ribs and belly) expansion, which is called "excursion," and when auxiliary muscles dominate. When this pattern becomes engrained, the diaphragm loses its dominance, and becomes "inhibited."

Here is where pace of breathing comes in: you now breathe faster because you have to, and this Vertical Breath is shallower by definition. Your breathing pattern becomes fast and unbalanced. Realize that "pattern" can be a confusing word, though it's the most commonly used term in respiratory health literature. What we need to include is the "style" of breathing or Location of Movement in order to clarify the process.

> Montreal-based Kevin Secours, Director of the International Combat Systema Association, who has been teaching mobility and breathing for decades, explained to me in a personal correspondence how continuous postural tension taps into energy: "A tense body lacks agility, and you need to be able to strike or shoot, without tension, using only the muscles you need. Even a small amount of consistent tension is a huge energy suck."

ARE YOU LOCKED UP?

Traditional medical literature considers diaphragm paralysis the result of injury, motor neuron disease, or phrenic nerve injury. However, diaphragm inhibition can also occur in people who have a large waist even if they don't identify with being overweight. The compressive weight on the body makes inhales and exhales more effortful, and thoracic rigidity that is self-imposed is an all too common modern phenomenon. In sum, the constant muscular or emotional corsets that make for lack of thoracic flexibility bear the blame. Many of my referrals come from people who have been simply told that their diaphragms are "locked up" (diaphragmatic inhibition). And all of them have one thing in common: a low B-IQ score—meaning their Location of Movement is shoulders and upper chest, and/or Range of Motion at the diaphragm is minimal.

Manual manipulation is an option, but *releasing yourself* through internal stretching by using the breath and understanding how your body works means you "own the change," and, consequently, it becomes long term. The key lies in recognizing that your goal is to widen the Range of Motion of an inhale and to narrow on the exhale. In collecting data of more than 400 patients over the last two years, Belisa found that imparting this information in a step-by-step process that combines both intellectual and kinesthetic understanding (psychology/education and mechanics/strength) significantly reverses or corrects this inhibition.

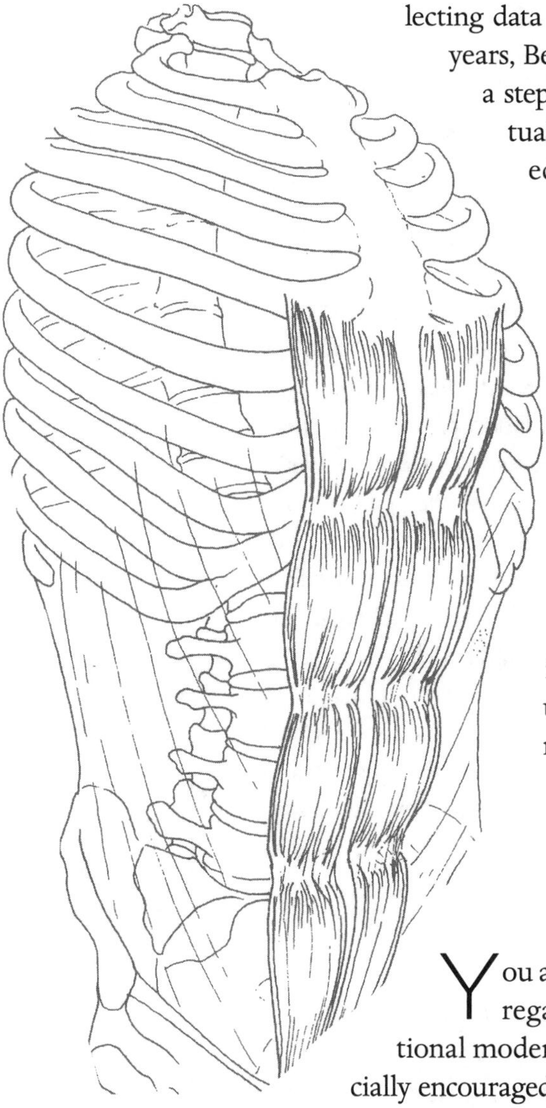

The "classic" pattern of diaphragmatic dysfunction, according to medical literature, is when the abdomen moves inward as the thorax expands during inspiration. Bad bad. The cause is accessory muscles creating negative pleural pressure that "sucks up" the flaccid diaphragm into the chest during inspiration. And here's the kicker: people are mimicking this abnormal pattern thinking it is correct. How much, then, is true dysfunction, and how much is underutilization because of bracing and misunderstanding?

WHEN DID BRACING BECOME THE DEFAULT POSTURE OF CHOICE?

You are probably bracing right now. Being "tight" regardless of your weight is part of our dysfunctional modern posture. This bracing can be an active, socially encouraged sucking in mistakenly assumed to be a good isometric to practice throughout the day, or a constant, simple tightness that goes unnoticed until pointed out. How does this translate to breathing? This rigidity of the body means lack of flexibility from armpits to pelvis. The breath moves up to the shoulders since it has nowhere else to go.

The consequent upper-body breath is shallow, and, because it's inefficient, it has to be fast to keep up with the needs of the body, which is why the instructions to just "slow down" the breath don't work.

Figure 3.3

Q: Why do I have to go from a belly breath to circumferential? Can't I just go straight to circumferential?

A: *Learning happens in steps. Your body needs the belly breath to unbrace. Running straight to the circumferential is too big a leap and you'll default to Vertical Breathing.*

Q: Unbracing is so hard, but I feel more alert when I brace. Will that change?

A: *Seems as if everybody wants to look like a superhero: big chest, narrow waist, shoulders puffed up with courage. Modern toy action figures have significantly smaller waists and wider chests, improbable dimensions for any child to look up to as a model of strength. These exaggerated builds (compared to, say, the average G.I. Joe of the 1960s) must have some psychological parallels. And while the "power pose" might be good for generating confidence before a match, it's not a great way to go through life. The posture inevitably forces you to breathe the most with the parts of your lungs that are the least efficient at exchanging gas: the top parts. Making matters worse: What happens if, after that big match, life continues to throw stress balls at you? Now you're walking around constantly braced. It's a power pose without an off button, a completely unnatural pose that should only be used in standoffs—attention all the time, or its evil twin, "totally disconnected." What does your "at ease" look like?*

YOUR STORIES

Understanding your story is important in dismantling your bad habits and getting consistency in your breath. And don't worry. Catching yourself throughout the day defaulting to Vertical Breathing is a step in the process.

"My dad was an alcoholic; when he got home after work the whole atmosphere in the house would change. I would hear him drop his boots on the porch. My mom would tiptoe, and he seemed to look for things to get mad about. When he'd start yelling and throwing things I would just brace my body and hold my breath until it was over."

—*Melanie F.*

"I remember thinking as a kid that it was good to suck in your belly, and 'good posture' seemed to mean tightening and somehow stretching upward, which I wanted to do anyway since I was short. 'Sit up straight' and 'imagine a string from your head' just made me tighten my body, and suck in my gut."

—Phillip M.

"My siblings and I would roughhouse, and either it was getting tickled or prepping for a playful punch, so I was always ready to brace my middle. When I was a teen I had an emergency appendectomy and felt like I had to guard that part of my body."

—Louis S.

4

THE BREATHING IQ: ARE YOU BREATHING INTELLIGENTLY?

If you take care of the machine—your body, both the inside and the outside—it will take care of you. Of course, you can muscle through until a certain age, but why not send yourself for a tune-up and make sure the mechanics are perfect (the muscles are strong) so that you are really optimizing yourself?

Research shows that by age twenty-nine your thoracic flexibility *and* lung volume peak. Which means that after age thirty, unless you are adding a breathing element to your training, the amount of oxygen you get into and out of your body is going to decrease—regardless of how much talent you have or how experienced your coach is.[1] So, if you are an athlete in your twenties, take note of how you perform on all the exercises in this book and keep working at them into the next decade. It's not chance that every person who comes to see me says, "I just feel as if I can't breathe as I used to." If you don't work on your breathing muscles and thoracic flexibility, studies show that your thoracic flexibility and lung volume will continue to wane. Can you get younger once you are in your thirties, forties, and fifties, and up? Absolutely. Read on.

If you do go in for a "breathing test" you might get a VO₂ max and some spirometry (FVC, FEV1). You might get told something

> You might remember as a kid going to your pediatrician and having them "palpate," or drum on your back (they were identifying asymmetries in diaphragm function). They also employed a hands-on-the-body test called the MARM, where they looked at how far their fingers moved apart on the inhale. If you were to go see your primary care provider now, as an adult, and indicate any concerns about breathing, they would probably refer you to a pulmonologist who by definition would focus on your lungs specifically. If you were to mention feeling anxious about your breathing, chances are you'd be referred to a psychiatrist or a yoga instructor, but neither would know how to tell you whether your breathing was mechanically sound in a quantitative way.

---

1   For more details, see G. Sharma and J. Goodwin, "Effect of aging on respiratory system physiology and immunology." *Clinical Interventions in Aging.* (2006) Sept.; 1(3): 253–260.

THE CUTTING EDGE

Rosalba Courtney is a Buteyko trained Australia-based osteopath with Ph.D. research into dysfunctional breathing and breathing therapy. Her Integrative Breathing Therapy technique uses evidence -based assessment tools such as the Self-Evaluation of Breathing Questionnaire (SEBQ) and the Manual Assessment of Respiratory Motion (MARM). IBT is a multidimensional model of dysfunctional breathing that identifies three key dimensions of breathing: biomechanical, biochemical, and psychophysiological. Dr. Courtney is a prolific researcher in topics from asthma to sleep apnea.[2]

vague about gas exchange and your lung capacity, and you'll leave with the information that you are "within normal limits." But rarely are you given tests of the mechanics with specifics of how to fix the deficiencies.

The first step, then, should be to look at the Location of Movement of your breathing (LOM). Next is to look at the Range of Motion (ROM) of your diaphragm. If this sounds a bit robotic and very technical, that's because it is. Your body is made up of a set of pulleys, levers, and hinges that are wrapped in muscles, tendons, and fascia, and the most important thing this machine does is ventilate, i.e., inhale and exhale. So, you should be asking yourself: Am I using my main breathing muscles and am I using them right? In sum, are you breathing "effectively"? "Optimally"?

HOW DO DOCTORS EVALUATE THE DIAPHRAGM?

Since the 1800s medical professionals have examined the effectiveness of the inhale and exhale by measuring different locations of the chest cavity. In his book, *A Treatise on Tuberculosis*, renowned researcher Henry Ancell instructed, "After a forceful expiration, and then causing the chest to be fully expanded, the maximum circumference should be noted. The difference is the mobility of the chest which is an indication of vital capacity."

Current research is peppered with studies looking at belly expansion, chest expansion ("thoracic excursion"), and both (abdominothoracic flexibility), and at how the mobility in this part of your body indicates diaphragm activity and, consequently, optimal breathing. The testing methods span from ultrasonography to fluoroscopy, dynamic MRIs, and nerve conduction studies. Many of these must take place in a clinical setting, can be costly or intrusive,

---

2   Personal correspondence, July 2, 2019.

or need lengthy clinical training. All look to encourage diaphragm movement.

The National Institute of Neurological Disorders and Stroke funded research that has developed a 3-D image "fiber grating sensor" that detects changes of approximately 800–1,000 bright spots on the body surface (Respiratory Movement Evaluation). A separate study conducted by researchers at the University of Hawaii and published in *Engineering in Medicine and Biological Science* used an electromagnetic sensor that detects chest circumference change by voltage output by focusing on measuring tidal volume. However, of all the techniques, the only one that's produced the most immediate feedback is measuring, from the outside. There have even been studies that looked at cloth measuring tapes versus metal tapes—an example of good reliability between examiners. Interesting to note that one of the largest studies to assess the efficacy of intervention/ respiratory rehabilitation had over 420 participants and used chest excursion.

Recognizing that modern life has added the stress response of neck and shoulder breathing, Dr. Erik Peper, whose focus is on respiratory biofeedback, added electromyography (EMG) of the neck and shoulders and the movement of circumferential, using a measuring tape with sensors (strain gauge). His results were published by the Biofeedback Federation of Europe.

The main point is that current research points to the fact that the more you breathe with your diaphragm, the more efficient breaths you'll take, the better lung volume, less pain, better regeneration— and the list goes on. You don't have to guess: take the B-IQ and get your answer. Track your progress and see your health and performance change. Abdominothoracic Respiratory Flexibility is the name of the game, which means the width of your inhale and the narrowness of your exhale.

What does the future hold? Imagine in the next decade utilizing an algorithm that shows specifically how your B-IQ grade relates to better balance, center of gravity, and endurance. We know that diaphragmatic breathing (ARF) is a key factor in breathing that allows you to downregulate, to get to that illusive anaerobic regenerative recovery state. Research already shows how diaphragmatic breathing relates directly to back health and injuries related to instability. Imagine how much more precise in-depth research will show the algorithm for a better mental game and everything that comes with it.

LET'S SEE WHERE YOU ARE: A SELF-EXAMINATION

1. ***Location of Movement (LOM)***: Where on your body do you feel the most movement when you breathe? What direction is it going in? What sort of a breather are you: Vertical, Horizontal, or a little of both, that is to say a Hybrid? Watch yourself or have someone else look at you. If you are puffing up your chest and your shoulders are rising, you are a *Vertical*. If there is no activation of your neck and upper pecs (you can see this yourself by looking in the mirror) and the only expansion is between your nipples to your hips, you are a *Horizontal*. Most adults are pure Vertical Breathers or Hybrids. Few, if any, are pure Horizontal Breathers without training.

2. ***Range of Motion (ROM)***: Measuring your "excursion" or "respiratory amplitude." Focus on two numbers: inhale, and note that number, exhale, and note that number. It's as easy as measuring a neck for a shirt, a waist for pants, or chest circumference for a bra. See below for the specifics.

HOW TO MEASURE

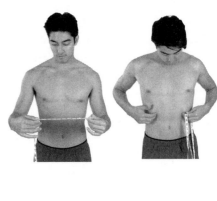

1. Find the bottom of your front rib (it should be directly below your nipple).

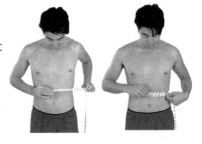

2. Loop a cloth measuring tape around your body at this place. You might find looking down cumbersome; if so, try doing this in front of a mirror.

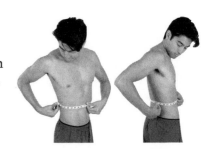

3. Holding the tape snug so that it doesn't droop in the back, take a measurement of the circumference on the inhale.

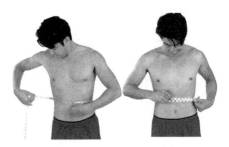

4. Keeping that tape snug, exhale completely. Take a second measurement.

DO THE MATH

First of all, is there a difference between the inhale and the exhale? There might not be. For some, it might be half an inch. For others, it might be two or three inches. Secondly, divide that by the measurement of your exhale (if this seems like a weird division to make, use your calculator). To have the number make sense, think of it as a percentage—meaning multiply it by 1,000, or move the decimal to the right three spots.

Remember, you have to consider your style (LOM) to get your grade! *Vertical*: you move up on the inhale, you see your auxiliary muscles engage. *Horizontal*: nothing moves on the top of your body; your belly and lower ribs widen on inhale, narrow on exhale. *Hybrid*: a bit of both.

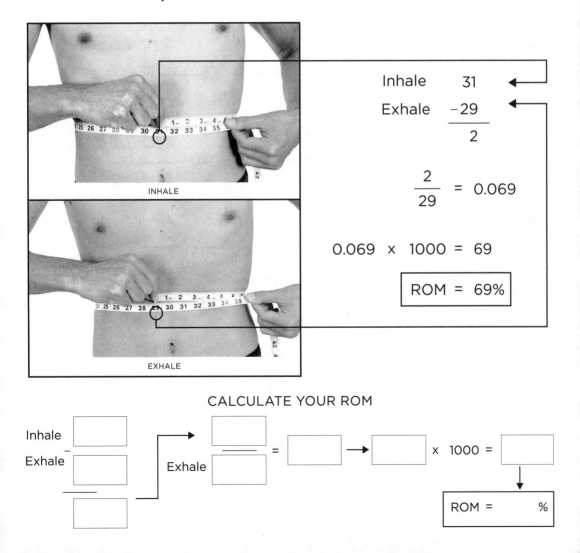

INHALE

EXHALE

$$\begin{array}{r} \text{Inhale} \quad 31 \\ \text{Exhale} \quad -29 \\ \hline 2 \end{array}$$

$$\frac{2}{29} = 0.069$$

$$0.069 \times 1000 = 69$$

ROM = 69%

CALCULATE YOUR ROM

Inhale ▢
−
Exhale ▢

▢

⟶ Exhale ▢ ▭ = ▢ ⟶ ▢ × 1000 = ▢

ROM =   %

Remember that your grade is indicative of two things: the Range of Motion (ROM) and the Location of Movement (LOM) of your breath. Your B-IQ grade will answer the question: Am I using my diaphragm? Got a "D"? Not so much; you have work to do. Got a "B"? Keep working toward that "A." Got an "A"? The answer is *yes*, so work on strengthening those muscles now that you have the mechanics right.

Here's the graph to figure it out:

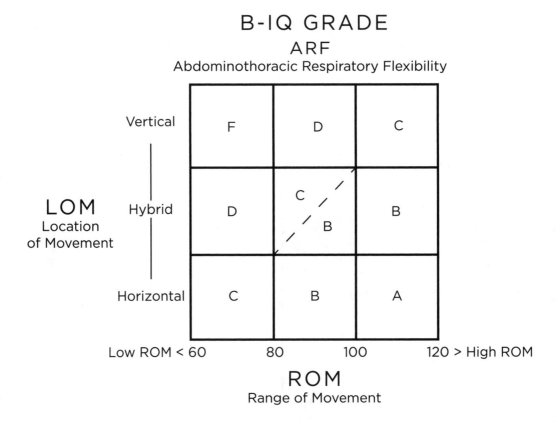

Hate math? Here's an alternative and simpler way to look at it.

SIMPLE STEPS

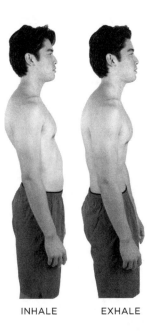

INHALE   EXHALE

Breathe without moving your shoulders.

• If your exhale measurement is 20 inches or greater, your inhale should exceed it by at least 2 inches. (In other words, if your inhale and exhale are in the 20s, there should be a difference of 2–3 inches between them.)

• If your exhale measurement is 30 inches or greater, your inhale should exceed it by at least 3 inches. (In other words, if your inhale and exhale are in the 30s, there should be 3–4 inches difference between them.)

• If your exhale measurement is 40 inches or greater, your inhale should exceed it by at least 4 inches. (In other words, if your inhale and exhale are in the 40s, there should be about 4 inches between them.)

For this simple calculation, you should be breathing horizontally like this.

EXHALE	INHALE
≤ 20 inches	+ 2 inches
≤ 30 inches	+ 3 inches
≤ 40 inches	+ 4 inches

YOUR STORIES

FOCUS ON INHALE OR EXHALE? CONSIDER YOUR BODY TYPE.
If you are lanky or lean you are going to want to focus on your inhale getting wider. If you have a few extra pounds on you, you will want to focus on your exhale.

"I'm tall and lanky; my exhale was a 30 and my inhale a 31. So, I'm working on getting my inhale to be at least three inches more than my exhale, to 33."

—*Will K.*

"I'm off-season and I'm at least 30 pounds overweight. I started at a 44 inhale, 43 exhale. I know I have to work on my exhale, I'm working on getting it down to at least 40."

—*Marell S.*

FINALLY: A FUNCTIONAL, MEANINGFUL
MEASUREMENT FOR BREATHING

Too often with medical testing, people get "results" but they don't know what the numbers really mean, how they affect their lives practically, and—most important—how to change them for the better.

Keep in mind that the B-IQ is a functional measurement, which means that it is practical, useful, and that it intuitively empowers you. Yes, you can, and should, take and retake the test, and track your progress over time. As your score improves, you can also evaluate the impact these changes have on your daily life.

The beauty of the B-IQ is that it makes sense. When you let your body widen on the inhale, it means your diaphragm is working: it's flattening and expanding your thoracic cavity. You are trying not to breathe vertically, because that uses auxiliary muscles that were never meant to be primary breathing muscles.

1. The first step in this system is to understand it intellectually (i.e., that the above paragraph makes sense in a way that it never has before).
2. Next comes the ability to visualize the parts of the "machine" and how they should be operating and interacting.
3. Then comes having the sensation; that is to say, the kinesthetic experience of what is right, wrong, good, and better. That lightbulb, that "a-ha moment," has to occur several times in the process.

The simplicity of this instruction makes for a massive reorganization of what you previously thought as correct. But listen up, because here's what's truly interesting: You'll start looking around you and seeing how much misunderstanding there is out there. Watch how people mistakenly gesticulate upward when talking about a deep breath!

DO THIS NOW

Right now, go measure someone else. Teaching someone material you are starting to grasp is one of the best ways to learn.

FREQUENTLY ASKED QUESTIONS

Q: Well, now that I know what makes for a better grade, I can purposefully not use my shoulders, push out my belly for an inhale, and narrow for an exhale. I know my grade will be better, but does that count?

A: *Yes. This isn't a test of whether you do it or not; it's a test of whether you can do it. But hang on: coming up next, we have to look at the strength of these muscles! So now think about the following. Say you get a grade lower than you were expecting, and you are surprised because you thought you were using your diaphragm. More than anything, then, your grade gives you something to sink your teeth into. It works as a baseline.*

Q: I got a good grade. What does that mean?

A: *It means your mechanics are good, that you are using your main breathing muscles and accessing the best part of your lungs. Your job now is to strengthen the muscles.*

Q: I scored an "A." Should I go on to the next chapter?

A: *Sure, skip ahead. This book is arranged so that you can open up, read, and work on different sections.*

Q: I have good expansion (ROM), but bad style (LOM). I keep using my shoulders. What's more important?

A: *It's better first to fix your Location of Movement (style), and then work on your ROM. So, keep your shoulders relaxed and focus on widening on your inhale and narrowing on your exhale. Depending on your body type, you'll find one more challenging than the other.*

Q: My style is horizontal, but the difference between the inhale and exhale is low. What's my homework?

A: *So, your Location of Movement (horizontal) is good, but your Range of Motion is not as good. The short answer is, stretch and learn to* widen on the inhale and strengthen your muscles to narrow on the exhale. For the longer answer, here's a question: Is it your inhale that needs work or your exhale? This is something that you'll be able to determine easily: your inhale feels wide, but the narrow isn't happening as thoroughly. Sometimes folks who are tight in the middle, are "rib grippers" (we'll talk more about that), or very muscular, and consequently have a hard time inhaling. Sometimes people with a little more weight on around the middle also have a hard time with the exhale. It feels like an ab exercise and they might break a sweat (and they should).

Q: When I fixed my LOM, my expansion, ROM, got smaller. Is this normal?

A: *Yes, and I bet your grade likely got better. Before, you were moving your thoracic cavity with your shoulders, so the expansion was happening by default owing to the fact that you were pulling upward. Now you are actually using your diaphragm and letting your neck and shoulders rest. Your diaphragm is pushing your rib cage open at the bottom, the way it was designed to. Your ROM (and grade) will get better, so keep practicing. (More exercises to follow.)*

Q: Breathing horizontally doesn't feel as satisfying. Is that normal?

A: *Yes, and it will change; don't worry. Think about when you sigh or stop for a moment to take a deep breath. Although it isn't a deep breath given the volume of air you are pulling in, you are pausing, loosening your body, and tuning in to yourself for a few seconds. Take a Horizontal Breath, relax your jaw and shoulders; your association with this breath will change, especially now that you know this breath is actually good for your body and is truly "deep."*

Q: I've been told that putting my hands on my waist, like a referee, and breathing into them makes me breathe diaphragmatically. Is this true?

A: *No; in fact, this posture makes people revert to a Vertical Breath, in which their shoulders jerk upward. If you do try it, make sure that your shoulders don't lift and your neck muscles don't kick in. In addition, this pose limits your attention to a "lateral breath," whereas what we really want is a circumferential one.*

Q: **What about wearables? Do they train the diaphragm?**

A: *Most new breathing wearables look at breathing patterns rather than at the Location of Movement or Range of Motion. While patterned breathing can be helpful in slowing down the breath, the LOM and ROM are far more important.*

Q: **Why such an emphasis on "no shoulders"?**

A: *Because it's hard to breathe without moving them—although it shouldn't be. Your neck and shoulders do have accessory breathing muscles but we want to see how much you can use your diaphragm as your primary breathing muscle. While you can expand your rib cage by pulling up with your shoulders, this means that your diaphragm is still not bearing its load of the work and, consequently, you're burdening your neck and shoulder breathing muscles. This upward breath is ineffective (needs more breaths to get the same amount of air than with a lower-body breath) and inefficient (it ends up taking up more energy than it creates, which, during competition, can be critical).*

Q: **Should I use my nose or my mouth for breathing exercises?**

A: *Regardless of how you breathed before, switch so that you get a different auditory cue. If you were a nose breather, breathe through your mouth so you can hear it. If you breathed through your mouth, close your mouth and breathe through your nose so you have a different sensory experience: hearing it inside your head and feeling air in your nostrils. Later, once you have earned an "A" and are used to the new pattern, you should switch to nose inhales.*

THREE EXERCISES IN SENSORY LEARNING

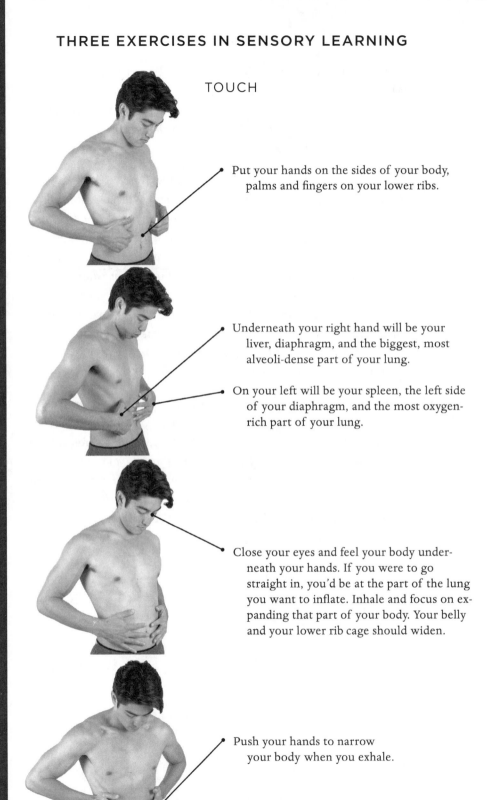

TOUCH

Put your hands on the sides of your body, palms and fingers on your lower ribs.

Underneath your right hand will be your liver, diaphragm, and the biggest, most alveoli-dense part of your lung.

On your left will be your spleen, the left side of your diaphragm, and the most oxygen-rich part of your lung.

Close your eyes and feel your body underneath your hands. If you were to go straight in, you'd be at the part of the lung you want to inflate. Inhale and focus on expanding that part of your body. Your belly and your lower rib cage should widen.

Push your hands to narrow your body when you exhale.

SENSORY LEARNING EXERCISES

SEE

To get a visual of what is going on inside, take a household metal vegetable steamer, turn it upside down, and flatten it (that's the inhale); now, make the edges narrow (that's the exhale). If you don't have one, interlace your fingers with your hands in front of you, palms facing down, at chest height. On the inhale, flatten your hands and spread your fingers. On the exhale, make the circumference of your hands smaller (think of the outer rim of an umbrella).

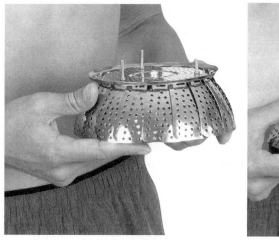 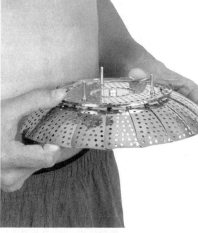

FEEL

Put your pointer fingers right on top of your collarbones and press inward. Here is the very top and the smallest part of your lungs, which has the fewest alveoli of the lungs. Yet these are the areas you use the most when you breathe vertically. This is why Vertical Breathers need several breaths to feel that they have caught their breath—they usually breathe faster.

So far, we've discussed the history and reasons for change and included your goals in the process. Let's move on to the fundamentals of how to breathe better.

SENSORY LEARNING EXERCISES

5

HOW TO BREATHE BETTER: FUNDAMENTALS

Here's a history from Belisa: Last year, a renowned pulmonologist made an appointment with me. Of course I knew his name. I had seen him on *Oprah*, when magician David Blaine held his breath for a record seventeen minutes. But I was sure he had mistaken me for someone else. Why would a doctor who had been the head of an internationally known clinic, who was a free diver himself, want to see me? I was sure he'd picked the wrong Dr. Belisa. My explanations must seem almost embarrassingly simple, I thought. I waited for him to laugh and ask if there was anything new I could teach him. That reaction never came. So, why was he here? In short order, he told me why: "No one teaches the how," Dr. Ralph Potkin said.[1] And then added, "You teach *The How*."

You learned in the last chapter that the crux of the problem with *subpar breathing* (meaning anything under an "A" on your B-IQ) lies in the mechanics—and therein resides the solution. This chapter will teach you *how* to breathe in a mechanically sound and anatomically congruous way. And, as I repeat in class, "You used to breathe this way (when you were under five and a half), and your body wants to breathe this way because your diaphragm is positioned in your body to be able to expand your rib cage."

This learning is unlike any other: it is a hybrid of intellectual, kinesthetic, and psychological. You can't see your lungs, or air, and the diaphragm is so deep in the body that you can't feel it. In sum,

---

1   Dr. Potkin is a Clinical Professor of Medicine at UCLA School of Medicine, and is the past clinical chief of the Division of Pulmonary and Critical Care Medicine at Cedars-Sinai Medical Center. Dr. Potkin was the team physician for the United States Free Diving team. Dr. Potkin is board-certified in internal medicine, pulmonary diseases, critical care, and hyperbaric medicine.

it's like a cross between physical therapy and a cognitive behavioral therapy session.

WHEN WELL-INTENTIONED CUES PRODUCE BAD RESULTS

When I first started looking at my patients' breathing, I found that when I told them to take a "deep breath," or "big breath," they would inevitably breathe upward, vertically. Their auxiliary muscles would kick in, rather than the primary breathing muscles around the middle. (Often, their midsection would even narrow, which is the complete opposite of what you want to happen when you fill your lungs). If they did widen, it wasn't much at all. Some widened in the front but crunched up in the back, or vice versa. This was true even for folks with specializations in anatomy, fitness, and health. Given my background in child psychology, I looked to see what beliefs or cues were causing this confusion and why. And I discovered that there's an enormous gap in understanding the components of the mechanics of breathing, although we all agree enthusiastically that it's very important. What I found were words, analogies, and instructions that were confusing, or exacerbated bad breathing.

YOUR STORY

"I thought I was breathing with my diaphragm; in fact, I was sure I was. Then we measured. I wasn't. I was surprised. But the numbers don't lie."

—Larry M.

TO GET YOUR B-IQ TO AN "A"

DIAPHRAGM EXTENSIONS

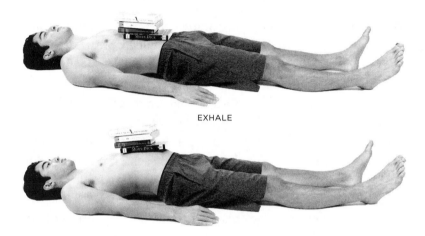

EXHALE

INHALE

ROCK AND ROLL

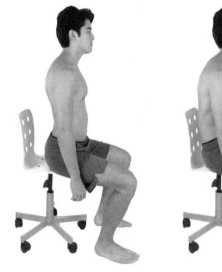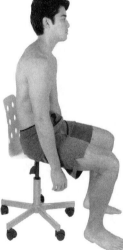

INHALE   EXHALE

TO GET YOUR B-IQ TO AN A

CAT/COW

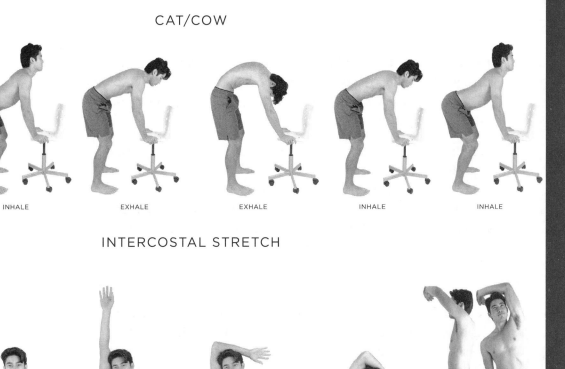

INHALE   EXHALE   EXHALE   INHALE   INHALE

INTERCOSTAL STRETCH

INHALE   EXHALE   INHALE   EXHALE   INHALE   EXHALE

Variation

SPINAL TWIST

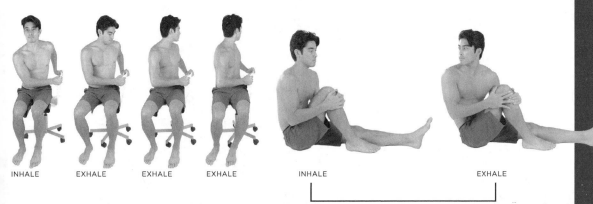

INHALE   EXHALE   EXHALE   EXHALE   INHALE   EXHALE

Variation

TO GET YOUR B-IQ TO AN A

FREQUENTLY ASKED QUESTIONS

Q: Tipping forward is hard only in that it feels like my hamstrings are holding me back. Is this possible?

A: Yes, and yet another reason you need to work on stretching your hamstrings. They affect your breathing.

Q: I am breathing but I have no side movement. My belly just pops. Is that correct?

A: It's on the way. This is a good first-learning breath in that it helps your brain understand that breathing has to do with movement in the middle of your body, not on the top. The next step is to start to get the ribs to move, both on the inhale and exhale.

STIMULATE. LOCATE. RECRUIT.

1. ***STIMULATE***. Take the very tip of your thumb and find the gap between two ribs anywhere on your body. Press firmly as if you are trying to create space between the ribs. Now inhale and exhale horizontally, encouraging a millimeter more of "give" at that point. Move your finger to different spots on your rib cage. Visualize these intercostal muscles in your mind's eye.

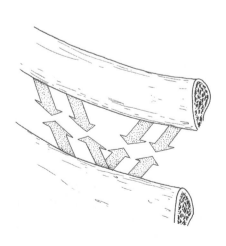
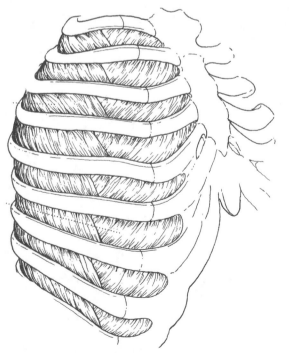

Figure 5.1

2. *LOCATE*. See for yourself. Make the shape of a small "C" with your hand. There should be about two inches between your fingers and your thumb. At your side, hook your fingers into your bottom rib and press your thumb into the space between the ribs. Now inhale and stretch to the opposite side so that you are "opening" the side with your hand on it. Focus on the space between your fingers. Can you get that to increase? On the exhale, see if you can contract that same side of your body, and have the fingers come together, into a smaller-shaped "C." Visualize these muscles between your ribs expanding, then coming together.

3. *RECRUIT*. Use a dumbbell (between 5–20 pounds depending on your strength) to help you open up your non-weight-bearing side. Holding the weight in your right hand, arm relaxed, inhale and let the weight of the dumbbell deepen the stretch to the right. Let the weight help you deepen the stretch on the left side of the rib cage as you inhale. Now, instead of just coming back up, bring attention to the muscles on the side of your body that is "opened," contract them, and use them to help you come up (feel as if you are "squeezing"). Watch yourself in the mirror to make sure you are staying completely upright due to the fact that the tendency is to lean forward. Do 10 reps on each side, making sure you pair the inhale with the stretch and the exhale with the contraction of your body. Don't let yourself lose focus and default to "just moving the weight"—you are doing two very different subtle things in each part of this movement. This will help your intercostals both stretch open on the inhale and get stronger on the exhale, and narrow your body. The goal here, interestingly, is to do this hard enough today to feel sore tomorrow. Most people come back and say things like, "I didn't realize how much muscle I had at my sides." Since respiratory musculature is hard to feel, we have to get creative. As you add weight, say going from 10 pounds to 20 or 30, remember that this movement is really a hybrid. Your goal is that the weight helps you stretch on the inhale: your rib cage on the non-weighted side should be "opening" and your goal should be

that the weight pulls you lower, deeper into the stretch. On the exhale, focus on contracting the same muscles you just stretched. You may find yourself saying, "I can feel this in my back."

> *In rugby, combat sports, or any sport where you are at risk for a rib injury, having the rib cage flexibility that we are building here leaves you less at risk for a rib fracture.*

REINFORCE ANATOMICALLY CORRECT BREATHING

1. Hold two kettlebells or weights (as if you were doing a Farmer's Carry) with one in each hand. Make sure your shoulders are relaxed. Let the weight of the kettlebell pull your arms down. You aren't going to walk with them, so you can let your arms relax. Note: the weights should not be so heavy that you need to brace your body. They should be just heavy enough that they serve as reminders to relax your arms and shoulders.

2. On the inhale, allow your glutes to relax and let your hips slightly hinge (your butt will go back, belly will come forward). All the movement should be from the waist down.

3. On the exhale, contract your glutes and let the contraction pull your hips in the opposite direction (posteriorly/hips under), and narrow your body. Do this several times, noticing the important nuances. Scan your body and check:

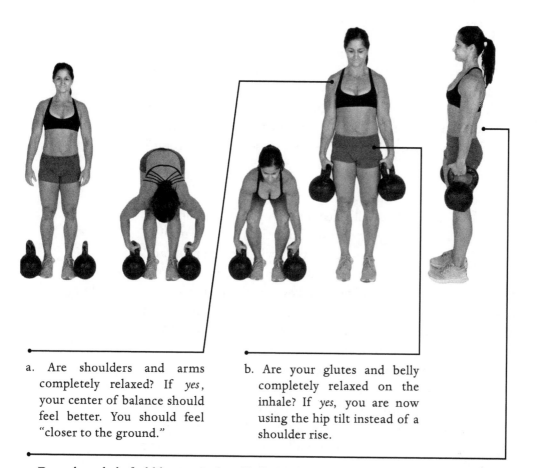

a. Are shoulders and arms completely relaxed? If *yes*, your center of balance should feel better. You should feel "closer to the ground."

b. Are your glutes and belly completely relaxed on the inhale? If *yes*, you are now using the hip tilt instead of a shoulder rise.

c. Does the exhale feel like a crunch, a "belly button to spine"? Once that feels normal, focus on your ribs and obliques, and see if they can narrow your body as well.

YOUR STORY

"I've always been fit but the last year I stopped playing basketball because of work, and Dad bod has kicked in and I have a bit more fat on my middle then I have ever had. So I've been sucking it in. It's only when I got asked to let it go that I realized how much and how long I was sucking it in. Somehow, I thought it would also make me stronger, but when I would let go and make myself expand to get my diaphragm to kick in, then I'd hollow

Model Tina Angelotti is the Director of Fitness/Krav Maga Worldwide HQ. She is a Cross-Fit and gymnastics coach.

out on the exhale and really narrow. I realized that my sucking it in wasn't making me strong at all, just sort of numb. While it was fairly easy for me to stop using my chest and shoulders and focus on widening and narrowing in my middle, I had to work on letting myself widen, and then my exhale muscles needed training for sure. My breathing went from a 'D' to an 'A' in a week, and now I'll start getting these muscles strong."

—*Jeff M.*

"I'm what I guess you'd call an ectomorph; I'm super lean and I run. Over the last few years I picked up the bad habit of running leading with my chest. I guess I was trying to open up and breathe better. Until I started reading about the mechanics, I never thought that this actually makes me breathe more with my shoulders. I worked on breathing through my back and a bit lower, and not only do I feel more centered, I feel like I have more energy with each breath, and that I can link my legs and breathing cadence better. For me the challenge was learning to inhale and widen. I realized all the tiny breaths I was taking were with my shoulders. Getting my body to still stay lean but be more flexible in the middle was my focus. My abs and the tension in my middle were actually holding me back. I remember trying to widen and it was like my diaphragm was locked up. I went from a Vertical Breather to a Mixed Breather, and from an 'F' to a 'B.'"

—*Xavier O.*

FREQUENTLY ASKED QUESTIONS

Q: **Why does learning one mechanical movement feel so different from learning another one?**

A: *With gym movements, you can take from others that are similar. In this case, you have nothing to compare it to. In addition, your brain understands but your body is lagging. Give it time and use repetitions to catch up. Keep in mind that it helps to breathe in different positions, throughout the day. Catch yourself, then autocorrect.*

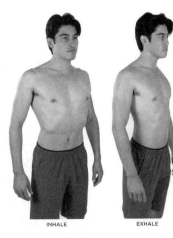

INHALE   EXHALE

Q: When I inhale, my belly narrows and my chest expands. It feels so counterintuitive to think otherwise. What is going on?

A: *This is an example of Paradoxical Breath. It is the exact opposite of the way your body is set up mechanically to breathe. You are going to need a lot of physical cues to help you change this. Put your hands on your lower ribs, palms flat on your body. Look down at your middle, inhale and widen, then exhale using your hands to suggest that the exhale is narrow. Adding hip movement to this will help tremendously. Be patient with yourself.*

Q: I keep hearing that I have to "tuck my ribs." When I do that, I stop breathing. What gives?

A: *You probably have what is called a "scissors open" posture. One of the best articles on this I've read is "Dynamic Neuromuscular Stabilization" by Clare Frank, et al. While tucking your ribs is something you should learn in order to help your posture and performance, you first have to learn how to breathe so that when you pull your rib cage to a better position (over your hips), you don't end up hovering or just bracing your upper body and holding your breath.*

Q: Can I ever breathe with moving my shoulders?

A: *Yes, if you are breathing hard. The problem is when you breathe with only your shoulders (auxiliary muscles).*

Q: Why does a Vertical Breath feel good, even if now I understand it's not really deep?

A: *One of the reasons you think a Vertical Breath feels good is that it gives you the external cue to calm down and focus inward. You feel your shoulders move, and you pay attention to the feeling of air in your nostrils and throat. Right now, try this: pretend you are yawning, open your mouth wide, flare your nostrils, and relax your jaw.*

Q: I can pop my belly, but then I feel stuck. What is happening?

A: *Belly pops start somatic learning of what breathing should feel like. You start to be aware of a sensation at your sides and grasp the concept of a widening breath. When your belly pops, only the middle of your diaphragm moves (by association), so the next step is to start pulling the sides of the diaphragm open. The sides of the diaphragm open by being pulled by your outer intercostals. These are tight and not used to working. They are being held closed by your bracing, your abs, back, and your emotions.*

RETAKING YOUR B-IQ

Now, to get your baseline. Start with a belly breath, then inhale without moving your shoulders. If you can get the sides of your body to expand a little, do it; just don't default to using your upper body. Most people do this out of a bad habit owing to the fact that their diaphragm is a little "locked up."

1. Have someone watch you to make sure you aren't using the top of your chest or shoulders. Your upper pecs may engage slightly, but make sure you keep the width in your middle.

2. Make sure that as you try to widen your ribs, you don't narrow your belly. The breathing we are trying to measure is abdominothoracic, which, as the word suggests, is the simultaneous measurement of the expansion of your thoracic cavity and belly.

3. Notice how hard it is to do abdominothoracic breathing. What does this mean? It means that, like many people, you've traded in the efficient Horizontal Breathing that you used to enjoy as a child for *subpar, vertical, accessory muscle–driven breathing.* You've heard of gluteal amnesia, the "butt's asleep" condition plaguing desk workers that leads to loads of back pain? This is like diaphragmatic amnesia. Your diaphragm has fallen asleep at the switch.

4. Now exhale, and see how much you can flatten or narrow your body. What you'd like to achieve is this: that your middle expands wide on the inhale, and when you exhale you narrow your body. Keep in mind that the exhale is not necessarily just a "let go and recoil." Actively narrow your body and take that measurement.

6

GAME CHANGER: LEARNING THE 360-DEGREE BREATH

Mind-blowing concepts often present themselves as humble pieces of knowledge that your average person would simply skip over. Actually, they are unexpected shifts in perspective that allow you to see a new landscape that lies just around the corner. Have you had that quiet a-ha moment yet, the one where you find yourself looking at those next to you to see if they realize the importance of the concept as well? To measure your progress in the kinesthetic understanding of respiration, check off the points to which you find yourself bobbing your head *yes*.

1. You have intellectual understanding. It is firm in your mind why the middle of your body should expand on the inhale. You have experienced that moment when you put your hands on your body, where the biggest part of your lungs and diaphragm are, and really, kinesthetically, understand that that part should inflate—widen—on the inhale, and narrow—deflate—on the exhale. You can see the diaphragm in your mind's eye, you can trace it along your body, and start to see if you can sense it. Are you there?[1]

2. You are attuned and "awake" to the process. You notice your breathing in different situations and positions. This new alertness is part of the learning process. Your brain has

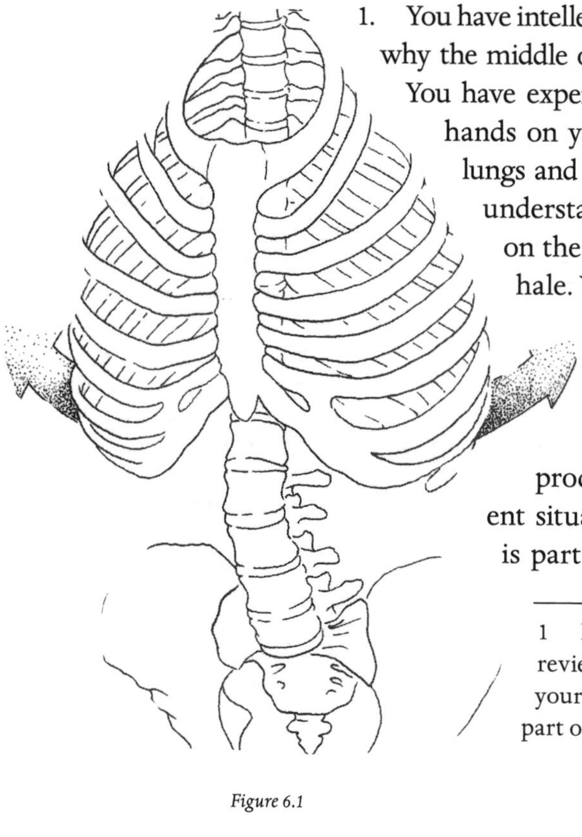

---

1   If not, before going on to number 2, go back and review the exercise on page 44 that mentions putting your hands on your body and locating the biggest part of your lungs.

Figure 6.1

new information and is integrating it. You pause. You notice. You get into bed and, before falling asleep, you are aware you're breathing in a way you never did before. Or you are in a pool or bathtub, or you are stretching the way you have hundreds of times before, but now you "feel" your breathing in a different way. You might find yourself "playing" with the breath, maybe even being amused. You can actually, subtly, feel places between your ribs and your back you never have been aware of before. Don't brush these feelings off, because there actually are some life-changing connections of learning going on in your brain. Quite to the contrary; you should nurture them.

3. You autocorrect. You notice how your default, braced, or numbed-out posture makes your breathing just "hover," or prompts you back to a dysfunctional upper-body breath. Now, when you catch yourself taking a Vertical Breath, you stop, perhaps berate yourself, and then autocorrect.

4. You judge. You can't help it, but now you are drawn to look at how other people breathe. You want to intervene. You feel an overwhelming desire to correct them and impart the knowledge that you now have. Don't resist the urge; jump in and teach. Nothing helps integrate and reinforce new information better than imparting it to others.

5. You sink your teeth into it. You find the topic of respiratory musculature enthralling. You realize that the little lung clip art you see now is such a visual understatement of what is going on. You know that over ten pounds of muscle makes up the machine that pumps air to your lungs. Breathing isn't an afterthought now; it's the infrastructure for both your movement and nervous system.

6. You spot dysfunctional cues. You notice how people gesticulate upward when

Battle Ropes Master Coach Aaron Guyett is an expert in wave physics and force vectors. He explains negative and positive postures in terms of "thrive or die." "Spiraling up in positive posture, consider the alternative posture, the one we are in while slumped on a couch (or nowadays, driving or seated at a desk). It may only be a few degrees but it's a comfort, to protect yourself from a cold position...it's the posture you die in, curled up in a ball. You can't breathe efficiently in that position and your whole body is hearing the opposite of thrive."[2]

2   Interview on April 27, 2018.

talking about breathing. You realize how mind-boggling and pervasive the myths and misinformation about breathing are. You can't believe how something so basic and critical has gone so askew.

7. You realize that all the mindfulness and talk of breathing to calm one down now actually make sense in practice. You think about breathing when in traffic, when you are made to wait, when you have to dig deep. You notice that taking a really deep breath both energizes and calms you. You really, really understand that breathing is the mechanism that controls arousal. You totally grasp the mind-body connection.

THE ADVANCED MECHANICS OF BREATHING

What do you do when your sport requires that you brace, restrict, or put your breathing in a compromised position? You should have the ability to breathe efficiently regardless. Advanced breathing means that you have a range of choices and breathing patterns. And you get this from a circumferential diaphragmatic breath—an abdominothoracic one—one that can rotate 360 degrees. Being advanced in your breathing mechanics means that you'll be able to find "a pocket of air" more easily when you are training in jiu-jitsu; that you'll be able to maximize breathing "through your back" when you are at the Hammer Strength seated row; that the weight of vest or gear won't negatively affect your breathing because now you are not using your neck and shoulders exclusively to breathe.[3]

As a coach, the more body awareness you instill in your athletes, the better their sense of

---

Many well-meaning adjustments don't have long-term staying power because they are done when supine, when breathing diaphragmatically is easiest. Once you stand up, your perspective changes, the feeling of what is right changes, and you are prone to defaulting into the familiar. The understanding that you are acquiring now means that you can actually help with the "adjustments" you get on the PT's table. And you can add to your store of knowledge by checking out the books of Bruno Bordoni, master of diaphragm manual evaluation.

---

3   A study published in the *Journal of Sports Science & Medicine* by M. L. Puthoff et al. found that "game tight" football shoulder pads impede the inflation of lungs during inhalation. Think about what your "uniform" is and how it's affecting your ability to inhale and exhale.

body in space, their precision, and their ability to back off when they need to in order to avoid getting injured. The body awareness that comes with optimal breathing leads to better proprioception and a center of gravity.

THE NEW FIGHT: LOOSEN THE DEATH GRIP

The self-imposed middle-body tightness that is deemed a normal part of aging is suffocating a sizable section of the population. And it starts early in life: research shows that the rib cage starts to tighten (and affect lung volume) in the late twenties. Then add to it the fact that modern man has never been as tight, compressed, and rigid as nowadays. So, while Donna Farhi coined the term "dismantling" in *The Breathing Book* in 1996 when describing how to start correcting breathing mechanics, twenty-three years later we have a new challenge: antagonist muscles that won't let go—tight exhale muscles, transverse abs, and intercostals that won't let you inhale, no matter how much you'd like to. Rehabilitative chiropractor Kathy Dooley of Catalyst S.P.O.R.T. cautions that if you don't "lose your six-pack" on the inhale, you aren't *really* breathing. So not only do we have to locate and activate our inhales, now we have to get the exhale muscles to relax and let that death grip go in order to let the inhale muscles work. It's a new conundrum.

If you can ditch vanity for just a split second and focus on strength, you'll realize that the expansion on the inhale will make the exhale contraction stronger because you'll have better Range of Motion. So, losing the six-pack on the inhale means that when you do flex, it will be stronger, more defined, and narrower.

Dismantling bad habits and using the right muscles requires that you recruit some muscles and relax others. Stop the tug-of-war between your inhale and exhale muscles. The juxtapositional force defaults to the path of least resistance; that

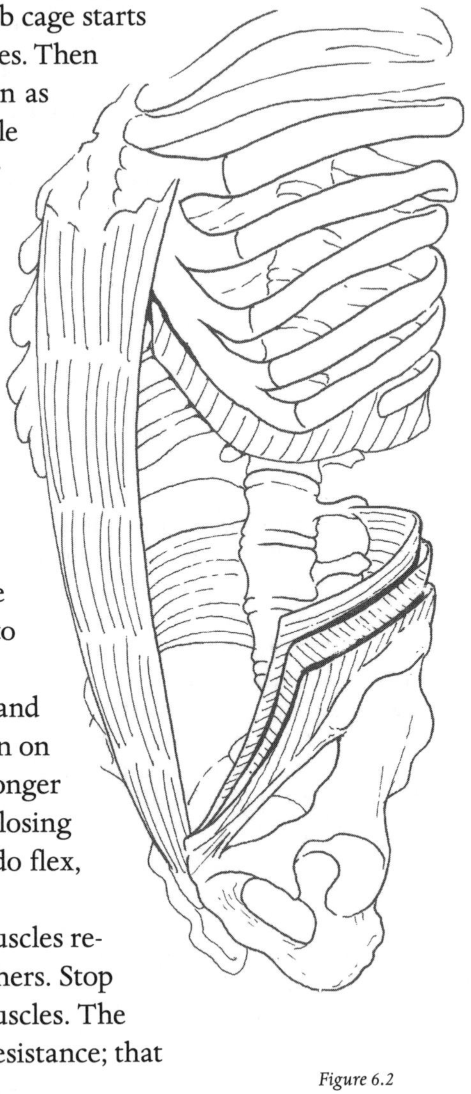

Figure 6.2

is, shallow, fast shoulder breathing or the opposite, none at all (hovering or intermittent breath holds). Activate your inhales by following my instructions and deactivating your exhale muscles:

1. Relax your transverse abdominis. You should let go of the muscles around your sternum, sides, back, and all the way down to your lower abs and hips. Notice the psychological and muscle tension that prohibits you from doing this. Work on it, going through one body part at a time.

2. Use the breath to stretch from the inside out. Lung pack (glossopharyngeal insufflation or buccal pumping) *gently.*[4] Pop your belly out; then inhale a bit more air (two tablespoons or so), and relax again. Each time you push your belly to be wider, the cural (middle) part of the diaphragm descends, making more room in the rib cage. Don't exhale; just remind yourself to relax. You might feel your intercostals stretching a bit. As you allow the air to settle, feel your rib cage expand in response to accommodate more air.

3. Pay "circumferential" attention. Allow the muscles under your armpits and the sides of your back to relax. Notice that when you redistribute and focus your attention on breathing in a circular way, you can feel a slight movement in your sides. In your mind's eye, trace the space around your body. You should be inhaling and expanding ever so slightly all the way around.

4. Redefine the exhale. Yes, your exhale is a letting go, but *only* if your inhale is truly horizontal. Most of us have gotten very lazy on the exhale, so give your exhale and narrowing some extra attention.[5]

DO THIS NOW

Take a Vertical Breath and notice how inefficient the exhale is. Now take a Horizontal Breath and notice how much more residual

---

4   See Dr. Ralph Potkin's article, "Effects of glossopharyngeal insufflation on cardiac function," in the *Journal of Applied Physiology.*

5   In his video series, Paul Chek says that this extra umph is "taking out the garbage."

air you expel. While you are learning, exaggerate the exhale. Imagine wringing out your body (or suctioning air out of a vacuum seal bag). Just the thought can help you activate muscles around your waist, and even on the pelvic floor. Also bring awareness up your back: the goal is to narrow your whole middle body as much as possible. You are now actively using your internal intercostals, which narrow your ribs and then squeeze the lungs underneath them. Notice that the entire muscular sequence folds together. Then, as you inhale, observe that it's a subtle movement forward. The diaphragm pushes the rib cage open; you have to allow it. Your belly is relaxed; it's widening along with your middle the way it should. Then your *internal* intercostals relax (you unbrace to take in more air) and your *external* intercostals kick in, pulling your ribs out. There is an effortless pause, then an exhale of breath, which is called the "natural pause" in precision sports. Now you have a "recoil." Take it up a notch and make the exhale more active. Lastly, let your *interior* intercostals kick in and squeeze your middle together. This feels significantly different from the simple ab squeeze when you started. Now you can actually feel the exhale at your back and the idea of a circumferential exhale makes "physical" sense. The whole sequence is a combination of opposing muscles that relax or activate, and when smooth, feels like a pulsating bellows.

BREATHING THROUGH YOUR BACK

BACK OPENER

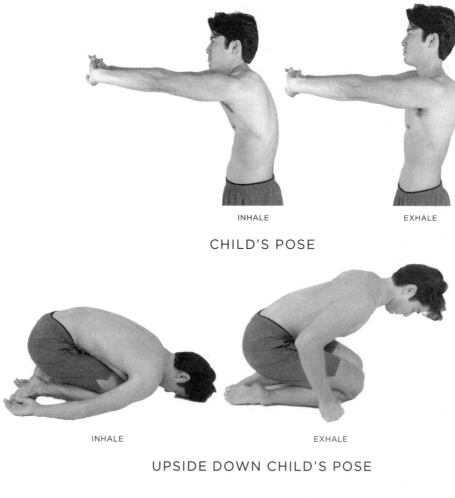

INHALE   EXHALE

CHILD'S POSE

INHALE   EXHALE

UPSIDE DOWN CHILD'S POSE

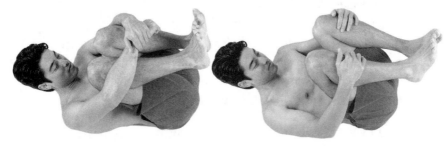

INHALE   EXHALE

BREATHING THROUGH YOUR BACK:
ACHIEVING A 360-DEGREE BREATH

With all three of these stretches, your specific focus should be on expanding your back on the inhale. This is a very subtle but important exercise. The movement is the smallest at the back when we breathe (as compared to the front and sides), but there should be a sensation of widening, however slight. (If you've ever done what's called "Crocodile Breathing," lying facedown and pushing the floor away on the inhale, this is the opposite.)

Most often, tight muscles and bracing make back expansion nonexistent. Having awareness of your back being able to move and expand while inhaling and exhaling means you are able to breathe while having a sense of elongating your back, not "crunching it."

Being able to back breathe is critical for sports that need flexibility as to where they breathe from: think of the posture of a cyclist, or the grappler as they shift into different postures while needing to be able to breathe from different "quadrants."

FREQUENTLY ASKED QUESTIONS

Q: I know this is odd, but I feel like when I take a belly breath it gets stuck. And when I try to widen, it's like I have a band around my bottom ribs. What is going on?

A: *It's normal to feel a nondescript but frustrating tightness that is limiting you as you work on stretching. Relax: it will improve with time.*

Q: Unbracing is so hard, but I feel more alert when I brace. Will that change?

A: *Unbracing and having a calm but alert stance may sound all new age to you, but it's something that Russian special operations have emphasized for decades. Bracing requires energy you want to be able to use. Inversions will help.*

Q: Will I ever be able to feel my diaphragm like I do my other muscles?

YOU'RE NOW ON THE PATH TO AUTOCORRECT

OK, so now you know what to fix. Think of it as when the yoga teacher "adjusts" your pose. Your mission is to autocorrect. And it's not as hard as you think, because you are just making your body do something that it's designed to do (and that you used to do well when you were younger).

"Breathing in combat sports is all about rhythm and timing. I remember sparring with someone who I'd block and strike back consistently. I noticed she would start the *sst* that came with the jab a millisecond too soon, and it would alert me. It was very subtle but once I caught on, the sound of the beginning of that exhale gave me all the information I needed about what was coming next."[6]

— Phoenix Carnevale, martial artist and fight commentator

A: You'll definitely become more aware of your diaphragm, especially at the edges where it connects to muscles on the outside of your body. You'll never get the localized burn you get with other muscles, because it doesn't have the same amount of nerve endings; however, you'll learn to sense and differentiate your breathing muscles by working out. What comes with it is golden: a better sense of control over your body and body awareness.

FIGHT CLUB

BREATHING IN QUADRANTS

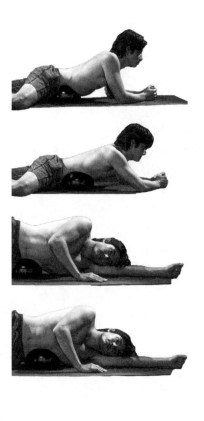

If you wrestle, grapple, practice judo, BJJ, or MMA, are a tactical athlete or just like to scrap for fun, chances are you are going to end up on the floor. Tough Mudders, Spartan races, and the like are also going to have you shimmying in the mud and holding weight against your body as you move. In jiu-jitsu, "knee on" is a position where your opponent will jam their knee in your chest, while "being stacked" is about creating distress because of upper chest and throat compression.

You should be able to breathe in quadrants, four in front and four in back. Using a Coregeous ball,[7] have someone lean on it when you are prone, and practice breathing "through" another part of your body. Turn on your side, with the ball under your side at two places, and breathe with your "other" lung. On your belly, have someone lean the ball into the four quadrants, one at a time, and breathe expanding in the three other directions.[8]

If you breathe only vertically, once the thought *I can't*

---

6   Interview on March 12, 2019.

7   Model is using the graphite Coregeous ball, which is available at http://www.tuneupfitness.com. Find detailed instructions in *The Roll Model*, by Jill Miller, Victory Belt Publishing, 2014.

8   As per conversation with Canadian pelvic floor fighter Smealinho Rama, May 22, 2018.

breathe comes into your head, you are more likely to panic (primal fear). If you know that you can get a mouthful of air no matter what position you are in, you'll feel secure regardless of the situation. The solution: practice discomfort or distress so that it goes from intolerable to annoying. There is the mental game element of being in a space that feels confined, which could be a result of your wrestling partner's attempt to smother you, or wearing a helmet and being in a small crawl space or in the darkness of a burning building. The same goes for pain, unless the pain is giving you information about an oncoming injury. Being able to discern and tolerate a range of discomfort means you are more resilient for it.[10]

> "Control your breathing or it will control you. Grapplers' Breathing is a deep anaerobic style of breath. The exact same as when you wake up in the morning. Deep and slow."[9]
>
> — Erik Paulson, legendary mixed martial artist, founder of Combat Submission Wrestling and author of *Rough and Tumble: The History of American Submission Wrestling*

EXERCISES

INVERSIONS

Assisted headstands against the wall are safe and may have several benefits.[11] In addition to a reboot of your nervous system with all the benefits for your mood and spine that inversion tables provide, they are a priceless exercise to secure your Location of Movement to your middle (take your shoulders completely out of the picture) and expand your middle (Range of Motion) because of the weight of the organs pushing on your rib cage from the opposite angle. Yes, you have to learn to tolerate the rush of blood to the face, which for most adults is uncomfortable because, unfortunately, most people stopped hanging upside down on monkey bars or doing cartwheels a long time ago.

---

9   Personal correspondence, November 2018.

10   Erik Peper et al. "The Physiological Correlates of Body Piercing by a Yoga Master: Control of Pain and Bleeding."

11   *The Wall Street Journal* published an interesting article on June 6, 2014, touting the benefits of inversions. https://www.wsj.com/articles/benefits-of-hanging-upside-down-1401747480.

In your mind's eye, think of what happens when you turn your body upside down. Your muscles now have to work in a completely different way. The push and pull of gravity are reversed, making every movement a new challenge.

You can use a FeetUp® Trainer or two boxes of paper, separating them just enough for your head to fit in between, and pushing them up against the wall. Your head should not graze the floor. If you need more height or they are too hard on your shoulders, add a towel on either side.

This position comes from yoga and is considered a safer headstand. All the weight of your body is on your shoulders, not your neck. Now when you breathe, you can't use your shoulders. Apart from working the diaphragm differently because it's now inverted, it gives you the experience of breathing without your shoulders moving at all (similar to the Farmer's Carry). There are several steps to achieving the headstand in this manner:

1. Situate your head and take a few seconds to get used to your head being down.
2. Shimmy your shoulders as close to the wall as you can.
3. Come into a downward dog.
4. Stay there for a few seconds.
5. Put one leg in the air, then kick up into the inversion.
6. Focus on how different the inhale and exhale feel.
7. Notice how you are breathing without any shoulder movement.
8. Inhale and let your ribs expand. Feel them move.
9. Exhale and include your ribs in the narrowing of your body.
10. Come down, slowly, one leg at time. You might want to stay in Child's Pose for a few seconds.

Leave this setup somewhere in your home or office. Pop up several times a day. Start using it as a muscle exercise for your intercostals, abs, and diaphragm.

Now while standing, close your eyes and try to get the same feeling as when you were upside down. Remember: inhale, you are widening; exhale, you are narrowing. Your goal will be to get an expansive breath no matter what position you are in.

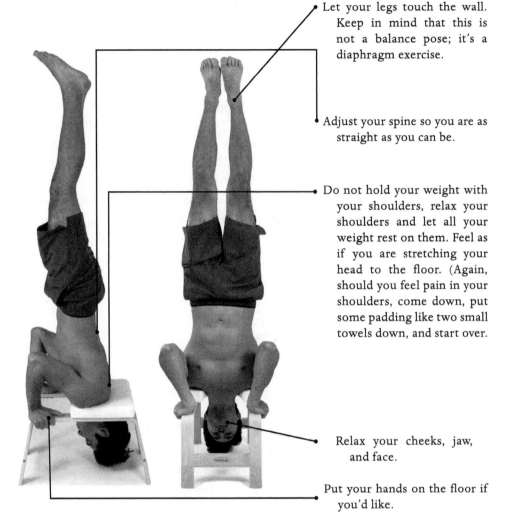

Let your legs touch the wall. Keep in mind that this is not a balance pose; it's a diaphragm exercise.

Adjust your spine so you are as straight as you can be.

Do not hold your weight with your shoulders, relax your shoulders and let all your weight rest on them. Feel as if you are stretching your head to the floor. (Again, should you feel pain in your shoulders, come down, put some padding like two small towels down, and start over.)

Relax your cheeks, jaw, and face.

Put your hands on the floor if you'd like.

FREQUENTLY ASKED QUESTIONS

Q: **I'm weirdly scared of going upside down during the inversions. What's wrong with me?**

A: *You probably haven't been upside down in a few decades, so go slowly. Luckily there is the "assisted version" that is better than a headstand for our purposes. Because you don't have to balance (you should have the wall to lean on) you can relax into the pose. That feeling of alarm will subside, I promise.*

Q: Does an inversion table work the same way?

A: *Nope, you can still breathe using your shoulders when on a table, and that is what we are trying to teach you to avoid.*

Q: What about hanging upside down?

A: *Same as above.*

Q: A handstand?

A: *In a handstand your goal is balance, so you actually have to stay tight and hold your weight. The goal in this exercise is totally different.*

A FEW DOS AND DON'TS

DO: Use this as both an exercise and a mental way to shake things out, to reboot your nervous system.

DON'T: Stay up too long at first; some small blood vessels in your face may be affected, which is minor and will stop happening.

DO: Go up often. This is the fastest way to reboot and get a real deep breath.

DON'T: Let your head touch the floor. If it does, you need to be up higher. Just get taller boxes or another towel to put under your shoulders for height.

STOP! TIME TO DO A SELF-EVALUATION BEFORE MOVING TO THE NEXT CHAPTER

Has your grade changed? Measure your B-IQ again and remember, you need to consider improvement in your breathing style as well. Has your understanding improved? You should be able to say *yes* to the following with conviction.

1. I am taking a breath that is biomechanically efficient.
2. I am taking a breath that is anatomically congruent.
3. I am breathing in a way that allows me to choose what level of arousal or what sympathetic state I wish to be in.
4. I am breathing in a way that supports my inner mental game, one that puts me in a flow state.
5. I am breathing in a way that pushes my strength and conditioning to the next level.
6. I am breathing in a way that allows me to really recover, to regenerate.

7

POSTURE AND PELVIC FLOOR: HOW TO NOT END UP IN ADULT DIAPERS

ANATOMICAL AND MECHANICAL BREATH

You may have heard that breathing can be broken down into two categories: an anatomical breath and a mechanical breath. Let's examine what this is all about, which one you should use and when.

1. *Anatomical Breath*. An anatomical breath is usually a continuous breath; in other words, inhaling is matched with the eccentric phase of a movement, and exhalation is matched with the concentric phase. On the inhale there is an extension of the spine; and on the exhale there is a flexion of the spine. If your body is coming together, compressing, then it's an exhale.

2. *Mechanical Breath*. A mechanical breath is when you manipulate a brace and/or intra-abdominal/thoracic pressure in order to lift a heavy weight or to help power a move using the exhale. Most weight lifting involves a mechanical breath; often there is a short, deliberate breath hold involved.

ANATOMICAL BREATH	MECHANICAL BREATH
Focus on if body is extending or flexing	Focus on spine and bracing
Fluid breaths	Use short breath holds/Valsalva maneuver to increase stiffness
Extending as you "open" or rise	Exhale words to create force
Exhale as you lower or contract	Exhale on effort whether it's pulling or pushing (whether concentric or eccentric)

However, there are times where there is overlap between the two: when working on a flow or sequence of movements you might switch back and forth between them. For now, just make sure you notice which one you are using. Do not default to a breathing style that does not support your spine when you need it, or to holding your breath when you shouldn't.

Be careful when using either one of these two breaths, because there are pitfalls. The biggest mistake with an anatomical breath is turning an overhead motion into a Vertical Breath. Even if you are raising your arms, there should still be a widening of the middle. On the other hand, the biggest mistake in a mechanical breath is maintaining a continuous brace, which leads to shallow Vertical Breathing.

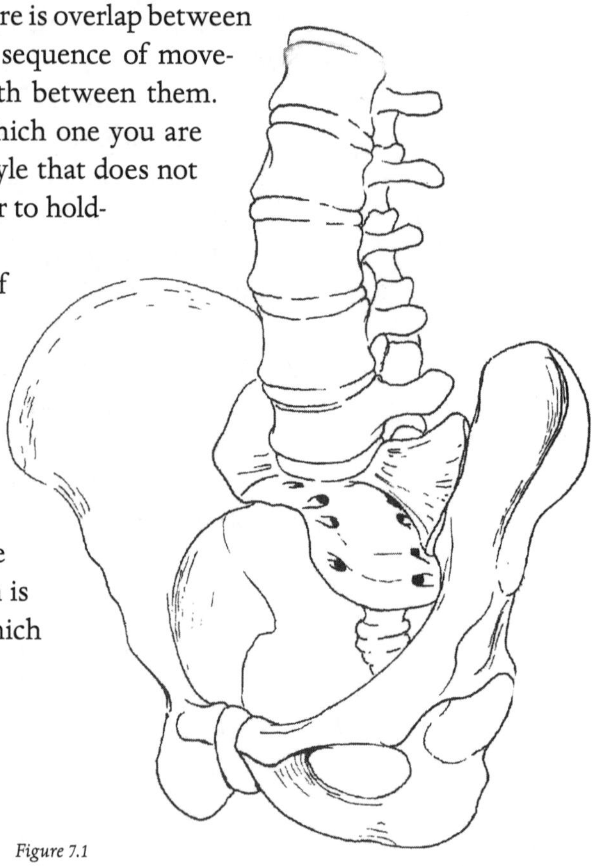

Figure 7.1

The alignment of your hips and thoracic cavity is a complex topic that cannot be done justice here. However, you should spend some time looking at your alignment, and your breathing is a key player in helping correct it. The importance of this is beautifully described by Ron Hruska, Director of the Postural Restoration Institute. Do check him out and his discussion of the ZOA (Zone of Opposition).

THE COBRA MUSCLE AND THE PELVIC FLOOR

The psoas is called the Cobra muscle by anatomy guru Tom Myers.[1] Let us explain: the psoas is what helps your diaphragm and pelvic floor work together. If your Breathing IQ isn't good, your psoas is suffering and being pulled or excluded (tight or overextended) from the process.

Think about your thoracic diaphragm as a soup bowl facing down, and your pelvic diaphragm as a slightly smaller soup bowl right side up. You achieve greater strength and balance if they are aligned one on top of the other.

YOUR STORIES

"Once I was able to visualize what my diaphragm looked like and how it was supposed to be positioned over and connected to my pelvic floor, I was so much stronger and felt so much safer."

—*Doug F.*

"Freakish Strength with Proper Core Training" by Jesse Irizarry (T Nation, March 2, 2012) is one of my favorite articles in terms of cueing and explanation of bracing and pelvic floor. It summarizes literature, gives you quirky cues you won't forget, and banishes some of the long-standing myths on the gym floor.

"As a dancer, the aesthetic of stretching upward and 'lengthening' meant that all the cues led me to hold my breath or hover. I didn't realize how this affected the fluidity of my movements."

—*Carolee W.*

---

1   For more on postural distortion, see his book *Anatomy Trains: Myofascial Meridians for Manual and Movement Therapists.*

PELVIC FLOOR: YOUR BICYCLE SEAT

Most people don't think about their pelvic floor until something goes wrong. What could go wrong? Well, less than optimal breathing (meaning a B-IQ less than an "A") can lead to, or at least exacerbate, pelvic floor problems. If you don't have pelvic floor problems now, statistics show that chances are you will. Everyone, it seems, is susceptible to pelvic floor dysfunction. Yes, even women who have not had children or have had C-sections are at risk for pelvic floor problems. And as a 2016 article by Ingrid E. Nygaard and Janet M. Shaw in the *American Journal of Obstetrics & Gynecology* points out, runners and weight lifters are the athletes with the most dysfunctional pelvic floors.

Often people already do have pelvic floor dysfunction problems but don't recognize them as being related to their pelvic floor or, as people do with anything physical that is not quite right, are just hoping and waiting for it to subside. If you answer even "just a little" to any of these, it's time to look up a physical therapist who *specializes* in the pelvic floor.

1. Lower back pain
2. Hemorrhoids
3. Constipation
4. Urgency or hesitancy to urinate
5. Hernias and/or diastasis recti (splitting of the connective tissues in the abdomen)
6. Less than optimal blood flow to the sexual organs
7. Pain around groin or hips, when sitting, working out, or urinating/ejaculating
8. "Leaking" when you laugh, cough, or jump

Be able to visualize it in your mind's eye. Your diaphragm looks like a large Frisbee. Below it is a slightly smaller one. Between the two Frisbees are your digestive organs and lower back. These frisbees should be moving in tandem with

"Being seated, whether in a wheelchair or desk chair, then adding a Vertical Breath, is the perfect formula for a poor digestive system and lymphatic congestion. But when we start rebreathing horizontally, deeper and slower, one of the first things that happens is that internal organs are finally getting the massage and pressure they needed."[2]

---

2   Interview on December 11, 2018, with Jean Baptiste, seated Tai Chi expert. See https://www.wheelchi.com.

even the tiniest breath. If this is happening thousands of times a day, you better bet that your spine, digestion, and even your mood are going to be better.

The second thing is to locate it in your own body. Feel the space between your sit bones, and front to back, between your pubic bone and tailbone. While the pelvic diaphragm is not as circular as the thoracic diaphragm, once you add the muscles that connect at the side and above, you have twenty muscles that make up the very foundation of your trunk.

And if that doesn't make your ears perk up, listen to this. Your balance, strength, and lower-back health are directly related to your knowledge and care of the twenty-plus muscles that make up and attach to your pelvic floor.

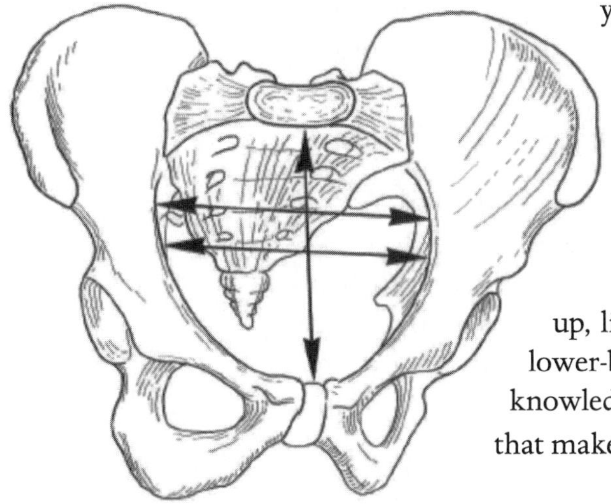

Figure 7.2

WHAT TO DO

1. Breathe using your diaphragm, taking a Horizontal Breath. Fixing the biomechanics of your breathing will automatically, positively affect the health of your pelvic floor.
2. Coordinate the inhale and exhale with the pelvic floor. Inhale and relax your pelvic floor. On the exhale it should feel as if it is squeezing and moving into your body. The relaxation during inhale is just as important as the exhale.
3. Check your posture: a constant extended anterior pelvic tilt means too much pressure will be pushing against your pelvic floor.
4. Co-activate and correct pressurization: When you brace to lift, include your pelvic floor. Otherwise all that pressure is heading down, to the path of least resistance. If you feel a descent or bulge (pelvic floor bulge) when lifting, you are well on your way to a herniation or loosening of muscles around your urethra and rectum. When you brace, you should be

co-activating the abdominals, *bottom*, and sides and back of the body.

The pelvic floor is not a smooth, thick muscle that wraps around your crotch and hips as any Barbie, Ken, or WWE John Cena action figure would have you think. It consists of three layers of tiny, intertwined muscles that have openings for your urethra and rectum (and vagina, if you have one). Why would you want to push down on it? Your pelvic floor reaches up to the front of the bottom of your spine. Just visualize that for a moment.

The most important takeaway from this chapter is an understanding of the amazing interplay of two very important things: breathing and pelvic floor health. Now you comprehend that the bottom of your body is intimately connected to the way you breathe. Grasping this concept will solve, not add to, another thing on your list of to-dos.

> EIUL (exercise-induced urinary leakage) is not a correlate of intensity; it's the beginning of a very slippery, very steep slope.

After reading this chapter, you'll know more about the pelvic floor than most people, insofar as where it is, how it moves, how it is connected to the thoracic diaphragm, and the importance of it being both pliable and strong.

As you inhale, the diaphragm flattens and the pelvic floor muscles lengthen in order to accommodate the descent of the organs. On the exhale, the organs spring full again, filling the space created under the dome of the thoracic cavity. Keep in mind the canister/soda-pop can image so many physical therapists use. Your pelvic floor is really the foundation of your trunk— the bottom of the soda can.

Don't forget the mechanics. If you breathe vertically (apically) as most adults do, using your

"RIPPED AND JACKED" . . . BUT BROKEN

Put together bad postural alignment and pressure in your middle, and you've got widening of the gap between the two sections of the *Rectus Abdominis* (or six-pack) abdominal muscle. The split occurs at the linea alba, the midline collagen structures of connective tissue at the front of the abdomen. Nutritious Movement Founder and biomechanist Katy Bowman is here to save the day, so check out her website and read her *Diastisis Recti: The Whole-Body Solution to Abdominal Weakness and Separation*—a book that should be smack in the middle of everyone's coffee table.

upper chest and shoulders, your exhale intuitively feels like a downward motion. Bad, bad: your pelvic floor is suffering because your exhale is misunderstood as "relax, let it go," and you're letting your body slouch downward. Not only does this result in an ineffective exhale (and retention of too much residual air), the consequent faster breathing pace is an attempt to quell that feeling of air hunger. The remedy? Train yourself to breathe right and your pelvic floor health will follow along with your newly acquired abdominothoracic Horizontal Breath. In sum, if inhale = widen the middle of your body, exhale = narrow. Consequently, inhale, relax, expand, and exhale means the whole "canister" exhales: the bottom contracts, the middle narrows, and the top (diaphragm) narrows the rib cage (by doming upward).

While research shows that many people make the mistake of bearing down on the pelvic floor on the exhale, in large part this is due to the dysfunctional mechanics that make for a downward movement of the exhale. Change the inhale and exhale to horizontal and a proper pelvic floor contraction makes more sense.

Q: Do I start with breathing correctly or addressing my posture?
A: Breathing comes first. Aligning your body correctly will come more easily once you have your breathing down. Plus, most cues to help with posture end up making a person tighten more, rather than relax on the inhale.

Increased digitization means that the stock value of paper media (such as books and magazines) has dropped significantly. What has taken their place? One of the fastest growing markets in the business is *adult diapers*, as reported by Market Watch on March 21, 2019: "Global Adult Diapers Market share to touch US $14.5 billion by 2024." This industry depends on people not taking care of their pelvic floors. (If they live long enough, all men will have some sort of prostate and pelvic floor issue.) And given that pelvic floor dysfunction is exacerbated by sitting too much, not breathing right, and incorrect pressurization of body due to faulty alignment, we are going to see the stock price of the adult diaper industries continue to rise.

HOW IS MY BRACING "BREAKING" MY PELVIC FLOOR?

Take a tube of toothpaste, undo the top, turn it upside down, and now squeeze the middle. When you brace only your middle (even if it is circumferential), you are "leaning" on your pelvic floor. And while it will take awhile, eventually it will start to crack and leak.

A TIGHT MUSCLE IS A WEAK MUSCLE

A tight pelvic floor to which you add Kegels just ends up getting tighter and weaker— and it's impossible to recognize from the outside. How to make sure that you lengthen? Lock the door and find a soft rubber ball.

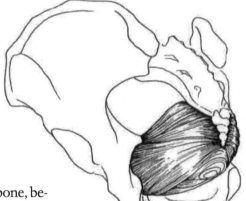

Figure 7.3

> *Step 1:* Grab a soft rubber ball and massage your glutes around the outside of your sit bones. Find trigger points.

> *Step 2:* Put the ball right in front of your tailbone, between your coccyx (tailbone) and your rectum. Gently lean into it. Move it to the right an eighth of an inch and do the same thing. Now you are on the inside of your pelvic floor. Move the ball slowly all the way around your "bicycle seat."

> *Step 3:* Now when you inhale, tip forward, and feel all the space between your sit bones and from your pubic bone to your coccyx relax. On the exhale, along with your lower abs and glutes, squeeze. Later you can squeeze it on its own without abs or glutes, and even finesse it into quadrants.

We'll talk extensively about bracing in the forthcoming chapter on strength, but for now you will activate your pelvic floor rather than exclude it, which would make it the weakest link and push it to herniate.

Sitting and Vertical Breathing has taken a toll on our pelvic floors. Now add to that the popularization of high-intensity intervals, weight lifting, and distance running with the body disconnected, and it's the perfect storm.

TRY THIS

The best movement to feel a rib tuck at the same time as a pelvic floor contraction with the breath is Cat/Cow. First of all, make sure you are going in the right direction. On the exhale, you are hollowed out, head dropped and relaxed, and back rounded toward the ceiling. This is an Anatomical Breath. On the exhale as you squeeze out all the air, add a pelvic floor contraction. It's a movement that will make sense immediately. Now, change to sitting up and try it again.

YOUR STORY

"Adding awareness of my pelvic floor allowed me to stay in a lower-body breath more easily. I added a pelvic floor contraction to my exhale, and a relaxation to my inhale (reverse Kegel) and I was able to 'stay low.' Plus, this is going to help my erection? Bring it on."

—*Tom R.*

THE RULES

Next, we are going to dive into breathing and endurance sports. But before you turn the page, make sure these three rules are at the forefront of your mind.

1. Make sure that, no matter what you are doing, the breath is integrated. You may be holding, you may be grunting in order to rebrace (which is what a grunt is), you may be exhaling on effort, you may be trying to add five more kettlebell swings. Regardless of your goal here, make sure your answer to "How are you breathing?" isn't "I don't know." Over the next few chapters, we will revisit this.

2. Make sure you aren't holding your breath when it's not neces-
    sary. Holding your breath because you are focused, stressed
    during a workout, or just not paying attention means that
    you aren't getting sufficient oxygen in and out of your body,
    which is going to affect your energy level. When you do hold
    to brace, do it right.

3. Between sets, breathe. Between sets is not selfie time. It's
    not "mull-over-that-last-shot-I-missed" time. It's a critical
    time—to decompress your spine, balance CO_2, and let your
    diaphragm and intercostals move to eliminate lactic acid and
    help you reboot.

We'll go through these steps in detail, with practical advice.[3]

---

3   Some amazing pelvic floor practitioners and advocates you should know
about: Julie Wiebe, Pelvic Mafia; Isa Herrera, Leslie Howard, Sue Croft, Mary
O'Dwyer, Tracy Sher of *Pelvic Guru*, Ina May, Stacey Futterman, Kathryn
Kassai, Amy Stein, Sue Kroft, Herman Wallace Institute.

8

BREATHING FOR ENDURANCE: HOW TO RUN FASTER (AND HAVE IT FEEL EASIER)

Long before endurance activities became sports—or a path to spiritual enlightenment—they were a means to survival. Humans were endurance running as far back as two million years ago, according to evolutionary biologists Dennis Bramble and Daniel Lieberman, who posit that endurance running is a derived capability of the genus *Homo*. The two researchers developed the endurance-running hypothesis, which states that humans survived and evolved because of their ability to hunt prey over long distances.

The idea behind their theory: humans are slower than most animals in the wild, and they lack natural weapons. They can't out-sprint a cheetah or out-muscle a gorilla; however, what they can do, in effect, is maintain a reasonable pace for a long period of time and cool their bodies efficiently thanks to their lack of hair or fur and to their ability to sweat.

"Everyone says humans are bad runners, because when you think of running you tend to think of sprinting," Bramble and Lieberman wrote in the journal *Nature*. "There's no question we're appalling sprinters, but we're quite good at endurance running."

Our ancestors used this staying power to their advantage in "persistence hunting," the practice of chasing an animal until it drops from exhaustion.[1] Persistence hunting would have provided our ancestors with a way to hunt long before the invention of the spear. There are records of this practice taking place in Africa (hunting kudu and wildebeest, as well as smaller animals), North America (the Tarahumara chased deer until they collapsed), and Australia

---

1   Email correspondence with Daniel Lieberman, November 17, 2018.

(tracking kangaroo). Interestingly enough, the practice still takes place among the Bushmen in the Kalahari Desert.

Fast forward to 776 BC, the year of the first Olympic games. The games took place once every four years for about a thousand years. The most accomplished runner during that era was Leonidas of Rhodes, who won the *stadion*, a distance of about 193 meters or, according to folklore, the length that Hercules could run on just one breath.

Halfway around the world, monks throughout Asia tested their limits along a (very) long spiritual path, with some powered by breath training alone. The Lung-Gom-Pa runners of Tibet were said to be able to run for 48 hours straight and cover 200 miles a day. A Lung-Gom-Pa in training would seal himself off from all human contact for nine years, living in a simple meditation hermitage.

> "Persistence hunting is the ultimate form of fair-chase hunting," according to Laura Zerra, primitive survivalist and author of the book *A Modern Guide to Knifemaking*. "While we humans are slower than our prey over short distances, we can use a combination of tracking and walking until whatever we are chasing is exhausted." (You can see Laura on Discovery Channel's *Naked and Afraid*.)[2]

If nine years of seclusion followed up by daily 200-mile runs sounds unbelievable to you, head about 2,850 miles west to Japan for something even more mind-blowing. There, the Marathon Monks of Mount Hiei would attempt to cover an 18- to 25-mile distance every day for 1,000 days or commit suicide if they failed. Since 1885, 46 monks have completed the 1,000-day journey, according to *Trail Runner* magazine. It isn't known how many came up short.

Meanwhile, on American soil, covering long distances on foot has a long and decorated history. Much like the *hemerodromos*, couriers in Ancient Greece, Iroquois messengers could cover 240 miles in three days. Apache warriors were known to traverse up to 75 miles per day on foot over some of the rockiest terrain on the continent. According to legend, a Pawnee leader known as Big Hawk Chief was said to have run 120 miles in under 24 hours—twice.[3]

The 1896 games in Athens marked the first running of a modern

---

2   Interview on January 6, 2019.

3   He also may have been the world's first sub-4-minute miler. US Army officers in Sydney Barracks, Nebraska, reported that Big Hawk Chief ran a mile in 3 minutes and 58 seconds in 1875, 78 years before Roger Bannister ran the first official sub-4 mile.

marathon, which at the time was set at 40 kilometers, or a bit under 25 miles. The first Boston Marathon kicked off the following year, with John J. McDermott of New York winning the 24.5-mile race in just under three hours.

The turn of the twentieth century was a busy time for big races. The first Tour de France took place in 1903 and consisted of six stages. The first and last legs of the race were each nearly 300 miles long. Around the same time, Norway introduced the Nordic Combined, a ski jump plus a 10-kilometer cross-country skiing race. (And if 10 kilometers don't sound all that far, you've never skied cross-country.) There's a reason why cross-country skiers have sky-high VO_2 maxes.

The first-ever Ironman Triathlon took place on Wednesday, September 25, 1974, when 46 friendly competitors squared off over 6 miles of running, 5 miles of cycling, and 500 yards of swimming. Among the crowd was John Collins, a Naval officer who adapted the concept, making it bigger and more brutal by combining what was then known as the 2.4-mile Waikiki Roughwater Swim, the Around-Oahu Bike Race (115 miles that they shaved down to 112), and the Honolulu Marathon into the first-ever Ironman Triathlon.

RHYTHMIC BREATHING: THE PROS WEIGH IN

Named The World's Best Coach by *Runner's World* magazine, Jack Daniels is one of the most highly respected figures in endurance running. He has coached eight national championship teams, produced 130 All-American athletes, and served as a mentor to countless other pro and Olympic runners. In addition, Daniels has brought running into his labs and studied it, step by step.

"In my many years of coaching college runners, we always had the runners record how they breathed and often tested them on a treadmill while running at different speeds to see what breathing rhythm they were using," Daniels reported in the Run S.M.A.R.T. Project. His staff wouldn't inform the runners that they were watching their breathing; they simply observed and noticed a pattern. "About 86 percent of them breathe 2:2," they reported. (The number 2:2 stands for "inhale for two steps, exhale for two steps.") And significantly, researchers at the University of Massachusetts, Amherst, confirm that while inexperienced runners have no particular breath-

ing rhythm, more experienced runners, whether they intend to or
not, will deliberately time their inhales and exhales to their strides.

"Most pro runners I ever tested used a 2:2 or 2:1 (or 1:2) rhythm
when testing them at hard workloads," Daniels states.[4] Why this
pattern? Daniels explains it has to do with maximizing a minute
volume of air, or the amount of air one can get into and out of their
lungs per minute. At a slower pattern—for example, inhaling for
four steps rather than two—runners can breathe deeply, but they
aren't breathing quickly. This can decrease minute-air volume,
since the runners are taking fewer breaths per minute. Conversely,
if the runners were to breathe very fast—perhaps an inhale on one
step and an exhale on the next—it would be next to impossible to
breathe deeply, and the tidal volume would be quite low. The runners would be moving air through their anatomical "dead spaces,"
such as the nose and trachea, which cannot absorb the oxygen they
take in. Daniels says his research consistently showed that for most
runners going at a hard pace, their minute volume of air was at its
highest when they were in a 2:2, 2:1, or 1:2 pattern. Note the words
"hard pace" in that last sentence. Daniels says inhaling and exhaling
for longer durations (three steps or more each) can be useful when
you are trying to run slower; for example, during the early stages of
a marathon, when you want to conserve your energy.

"Measuring effort through rhythmic breathing puts you directly in touch with your body, provides immediate feedback, and
gives you complete control over your effort and pace," writes Budd
Coates, a running coach and four-time qualifier for the US Olympic
Marathon Trials. In his book *Running On Air*, Coates recommends
employing a slightly different pattern, one that synchronizes with
an odd number of steps; for example, inhaling for three steps, then
exhaling for two, a total of five foot strikes. This is known as a
5-count (or 3:2) pattern. Using an odd number ensures that you
aren't constantly exhaling while landing on the same foot. The impact forces on your body are the greatest when your foot strikes the
ground. "If that impact is at the beginning of an exhalation, it
catches us at the most unstable times for the pelvis and core," ex-

---

4   Email correspondence with Daniels, September 10, 2018.

plains Albert Rizzo, MD, FACP, FACCP, in an American Lung Association blog. By spreading those forces evenly across your body, varying on which foot your exhale comes, you decrease your likelihood of injury.

BREATHING PATTERNS AND PACING: NOT ONE SIZE FITS ALL

Rhythmic breathing can also serve as an inner speedometer, allowing runners to measure their pace and adjust if it's either too easy or too hard. If they find a 2:2 or 3:2 pattern effortless, that's an indicator that they can run faster; that is to say, they can push the pace. If they're struggling to maintain the rhythm, it's a sign that they're going too fast. The solution: slow down until breath and footsteps resync.

Daniels says monitoring breathing is a useful tool to have in many situations, including when training above sea level. Runners will ask, "How much slower should I run up here at altitude?" And he'll answer, "Well, let your breathing tell you. If you use this rhythm at sea level, use that same rhythm at altitude and it will be associated with a little slower speed. And if you can't hold that rhythm, you're going too fast."

If breathing serves as your inner speedometer, then breathing patterns are like the gears of your car. As your breathing muscles get stronger, watch how your switch to a hard effort comes later. You can then shift between "gears" based on how fast or slow you want to go.

5:5	Very slow, relaxed efforts (5 steps to inhale, 5 steps to exhale)
4:4	
3:3 3:2	Easy running to long tempo runs
2:2	
2:1	Hard efforts, intervals, uphill running

Coates recommends the 3:2 pattern for easy to moderate efforts. For faster runs, one can ratchet up to a 3-count (or 2:1) pattern. He also recommends that runners experiment with the patterns in training to discover what works best for them (e.g., a shorter pattern is helpful when running uphill).

DO THIS NOW

Daniels says: "Run five laps around the track. First lap, do 4:4 (inhale for 4 steps, exhale for 4). Second lap, do 3:3. Third lap, 2:2. Fourth lap, 1:1. Then on the fifth lap go back to 4:4. And you decide which fits best."

YOUR STORY

"I would start my runs with four steps to inhale and four to exhale. I knew exactly when in my run I'd go to three steps inhale, two exhale, and at a hill at the end I'd be at 2:2 and 2:1. I worked on changing my breathing mechanics and strengthening the muscles, and that moment where I had to crank things up didn't come for another mile. I thought it was a fluke until I did it the second time. Nothing about my running had changed, just the breathing exercises."

—*Wayne R.*

VO$_2$ MAX: WHAT IS IT?

VO$_2$ max[5] is a gauge of your ability to supply your body with oxygen; that is to say, the maximum rate of oxygen consumption when doing exercise of increasing intensity. The rate takes into account every step in the process necessary for fueling your muscles, from inhaling the air into the lungs, to diffusing it into the bloodstream, to shuttling it through the blood to the muscles, to the uptake into the muscles themselves. A high VO$_2$ max is considered the gold standard for endurance athletes. Keep in mind: a high VO$_2$ max is not the be-all, end-all of performance. "I've been beaten by others with lower oxygen uptake over the years," says Oskar Svendsen, a Norwegian cyclist who scored the highest recorded VO$_2$ max to date (97.5 milliliters of oxygen per kilogram of body mass per minute), when interviewed by *The Globe* in 2014. Studies show that training your breathing muscles will not necessarily increase your VO$_2$ max; however, what it does is something better. Stronger respiratory muscles decrease your perception of effort and delay the onset of fatigue, allowing you to maintain a higher workload for a longer duration, which is the whole goal of increasing your VO$_2$ max in the first place. So, what's the takeaway? Train to improve your VO$_2$ max and your breathing muscles. Most experts agree the best training techniques for improving your VO$_2$ max are to run at a hard effort for between four and eight minutes. Try a 4 x 1000-meter run (about two and a half laps around a track for each leg) with two to three minutes recovery between each. A study published in 2016 in *Medicine & Science in Sports & Exercise* found this workout increased participants' VO$_2$ maxes by about 10 percent after six weeks.

NOTABLE VO$_2$ MAXES

- Highest VO$_2$ max (Animal): Iditarod Sled Dogs, 200
- Highest VO$_2$ max (Human): Oskar Svendsen, Cyclist, 97.5
- Average sedentary male: 45
- Average sedentary female: 39

---

5   To clarify: "V" stands for volume, "O$_2$" is for oxygen, and "max" is for maximum.

TARGETED BREATHING
FOR ENDURANCE

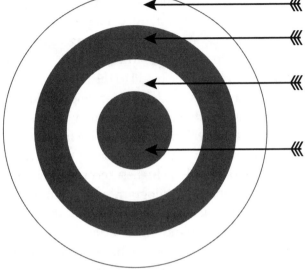

You are purposefully using the breath to detox, to heal, and rest.

It's the time when you're using your breath to calm your nerves and settle any pre-race jitters. Nasal only.

During this period, you are semi-conscious of your breath, checking in with it as an indicator of your exertion level, and making adjustments up or down in your pace. You may be switching to nasal in, mouth out.

Breath is nasal buccal (air coming in and going out of both mouth and nose). The sound of your breathing drowns out any thought. While the exertion is hard, you feel challenged but strong, you are in the zone, and have the goal in sight.

This target has to do with the awareness of your breath, given a certain moment of your endurance sport. Knowing how much you should be paying attention to your breathing will help with the "gear" and the pacing. First and foremost, you should be breathing efficiently, using your primary breathing muscles. Then it depends on the part of the circle you are in.

The bull's-eye is when you are breathing in and out through your nose and mouth. The goal is in sight. It's the only thing you are thinking about.

The first circle from the bull's-eye, you are adjusting your breath and the rhythm of your movement.

The second circle from the bull's-eye, right before you start, breathing is all nasal.

Last circle out is active recovery time; you are using breathing exercises to detox your body.

BREATHING FOR ENDURANCE IN A WEIGHTED VEST
(OR A BULLETPROOF ONE)

Anyone who's ever strapped on a weighted vest, or a 5.11 plate carrier in high-intensity interval training, knows breathing can be a challenge. Winnipeg-based Director of Sports Science and Performance at The Rink, Dr. Jeff Leiter, who trains hockey players and uses weighted vests as a breathing tool, told us, "When you inhale, you'll feel some resistance from the weight and the straps from every direction. It's an in-depth way to learn modes of lower-body and 360-degree breathing. Practice inhaling and directing your breath toward different parts of your body: your back, your sides, and your lower belly. Then try to breathe into all of those places at once, evenly."[6]

A weighted vest actually poses two challenges for your breathing: First, it places extra weight on the muscles of the chest that contribute to breathing, particularly during the inhalation phase of respiration. Second, the tightness of the vest and straps restrict movement of the chest cavity. Getting a proper fit is indispensable. "As a general rule of thumb, it should be difficult, but not impossible, to slide your full hand underneath the vest," says Brock Christopher, CPT and strength coach at Atlanta's Porsche Human Performance Suite powered by EXOS. "You want it tight enough so that it doesn't move around while doing dynamic activity but still provides comfort," he explains.[7]

> ### WHAT IS A "METABOLIC CART"?
>
> A metabolic cart is a computer on top of a set of complex machinery that's adorned with a lot of airway tubes—and it does in fact look like a cart. The machine compares how much oxygen is present in the room's air compared to how much is present in a person's exhalation. The difference tells you how much oxygen the person is utilizing. The data will indicate the amount of oxygen uptake (VO_2) and pulmonary ventilation (VE).

FREQUENTLY ASKED QUESTIONS

Q: What about patterned breathing for calming. Is this similar?

A: *No, slow patterned breathing for calming is different than this rhyth-*

---

6   Personal communication, March 28, 2018.

7   Rodio, Michael, "The Weight Vest Workout," *Men's Journal*, American Media Inc. mensjournal.com/health-fitness/weight-vest-workout/

mic breathing practiced with an endurance sport. So, you should be starting to pair a mechanically sound Horizontal Breath with a breathing pattern that supports your running (or with whichever endurance sport that has a rhythm).

Coming up next: there is deep science in how breathing muscle training improves endurance. We'll get you training them ASAP.

9

GETTING STRONGER, GOING LONGER: EXERCISES TO IMPROVE ENDURANCE

Have you experienced an intense but fleeting sense of fatigue while exercising? Being tired is exhaustion that lasts; feeling tired is being winded momentarily. And this temporary fatigue that you feel when breathing muscles are weak has a word: metaboreflex, which, despite having been in the scientific literature for decades, is still not referenced in the gym or in training. It sounds like a dinosaur or perhaps a supplement to enhance your metabolism. And since there haven't been instructions on how to deal with temporary fatigue until now, we've been sweeping it under the rug and focusing on cardio, which is simpler to understand than how to deal with training breathing muscles. A. Sheel, in the *American Journal of Physiology-Heart and Circulatory Physiology*, sums it up succinctly for us: "Metaboreflex refers to a condition when the diaphragm is fatigued, and, as a result, the body reduces blood flow to the legs (vasoconstriction, which lowers the blood flow to your arms and legs thereby providing more blood to working muscles in your core)." The good news is that you can train to delay the onset of the heavy feelings in your arms and legs. Strengthen your breathing muscles with respiratory exercises, and the heavy feeling in your limbs will occur later on in your workout.

To help you understand the difference, here are two symptoms of undertrained breathing muscles.

1. A heaviness in your arms and legs that makes you slow down, owing to the fact that blood is being drawn away from your extremities in order to power your breathing muscles. Breathing muscles that are "in shape" and trained need less oxygen.
2. A perplexing feeling of fatigue that seems to feel more psy-

chological (related to motivation, heart, willpower, or focus) than physical but is, in fact, purely physical. Since you can't feel your breathing muscles burn or tire the way external muscles do, it just feels as if you "don't want it bad enough."

There is substantial research documenting that breathing muscle training improves endurance.[1] And sports scientists have looked at IMT (inspiratory muscle training) with cyclists, swimmers, and runners, and discovered that, without a doubt, training the breathing muscles means better times and longer distances. In sum, the studies report that when breathing muscles are trained, they fatigue later and require less oxygen. This translates into feeling less heaviness physically, and psychologically more feeling of flow, regardless of the sport-specific training involved.

> Take two athletes, same weight, talent, training. The one who works out their breathing muscles will have better endurance and conditioning than the other.

YOUR STORY

"My heart felt like it was bursting out of my chest, my lungs felt like they were burning, and my brain was screaming 'stop.' I would go from focused and intense, to trying to find anger to motivate myself."

—*Omar W.*

---

1   For example: "Specificity and Reversibility of Inspiratory Muscle Training," *Medicine & Science in Sports & Exercise* 35, no. 2 (2003): 237–44; "The Effect of Inspiratory Muscle Training on High-Intensity, Intermittent Running Performance to Exhaustion," *Applied Physiology, Nutrition, and Metabolism* 33 (2008): 671–81; "Effects of Inspiratory Muscle Training on Time-Trial Performance in Trained Cyclists," *Journal of Sports Sciences* 20, no. 7 (2002): 547–90; "Inspiratory Muscle Training Improves 100 and 200 m Swimming Performance," *European Journal of Applied Physiology* 108 (2010): 505; "Inspiratory Muscle Training, Altitude, and Arterial Oxygen Desaturation: A Preliminary Investigation," *Aviation, Space, and Environmental Medicine* 81 (2010): 498–501.

YOUR WORST ENEMY

Your biggest enemy is yourself, but not in the way you've been told. Specifically, your biggest enemy is tired and undertrained breathing muscles. When they tire it feels as if you are lacking motivation. Next time you are gasping for air, waiting for the burn and sensation of cement legs to leave your body, rather than berating yourself, remember this: it's time to adjust your training because there is a new paradigm on the horizon. Since you are now training your breathing muscles, you can look forward to having better endurance, faster recovery, and you will find "flow" more consistently.

BREATHING: BIOMECHANICS AND STRENGTH

When you think about conditioning and endurance you think of running, maybe with a sandbag or weighted vest. You think of paddling out against the waves, five rounds of fighting, biking, running up stairs, or whatever timed running/lifting/climbing event you participate in. Whether you are a runner, swimmer, or cyclist, endurance athletes of all stripes live by a simple rule: The more efficient you are, the farther you can go. Just when walking around you breathe about 15 times per minute, inhaling around 12 liters of air. When you exercise, the demand goes up to about 100 liters of air per minute, and it may take 60 inhales (or more) to get it.

When you breathe, then, there is a lot more muscle than you realize working harder than you've imagined—and it's not just the 11-ounce fist-size muscle that is your heart.

Next, let's talk strength and biomechanics. Any muscle that connects to your rib cage can influence your breathing. The inhale muscles all expand the thoracic cavity, while exhale muscles compress it. When these muscles are strong and work as they are intended to, you get ideal results: maximum oxygen for minimum effort.

A 2013 meta-analysis of twenty-one studies led by Bahareh Haj Ghanbari and his team of

> "Johnny counted himself out in the third—just lay back on the ropes and gestured, 'No more' to the referee...I was angry with John at first, although I knew the line of fear and exhaustion he was walking. He wasn't hurt at all, just completely out of breath, and I knew within twenty seconds he was going to be wondering why he had quit like that."
>
> —*A Fighter's Heart*, Sam Sheridan

researchers at the University of Toronto showed that strengthening breathing muscles through training improved performance in endurance sports like running, swimming, and cycling. It documented that the strength of your breath is directly related to how far the diaphragm can move, or how forcefully it can contract. Simply put: stronger diaphragm equals more air in, more easily.

In 2013, Dr. Mitch Lomax, an exercise physiologist at the University of Portsmouth, ran a study of 14 mountaineers trekking through Nepal toward the 27,766-foot Makalu, the world's fifth-highest peak. Half of them performed inspiratory muscle training (IMT) exercises before embarking on the expedition, while half did not. By the time the climbers reached base camp at 16,000 feet, there were noticeable differences in arterial oxygen saturation between the two groups. Those who had not performed IMT had 20 percent less oxygen coursing through their circulatory system, but those who had done IMT in advance were only 14 percent desaturated, reported Lomax in the *Journal of Sports Science & Medicine*.

> ## HANDS ON YOUR HEAD OR LEANING OVER?
>
> If you just need to catch your breath, lean over. In an article in the *Journal of the American College of Sports Medicine*, researcher Joana Michaelson reports that, "The reason is that when you put your hands on your knees (or lean up against something), your diaphragm stops being a postural muscle for a second and can fully expand and contract with its only priority being to take a breath. The lean forward helps unbrace your body, take a fuller inhale, and slow down your breathing."

Researchers call the part of your brain that is constantly calculating what is a safe level of exertion for your body the "central governor." The idea was first proposed by the aforementioned exercise scientist A. V. Hill, and had recently gained renewed interest thanks to the work of Tim Noakes, of the University of Cape Town in South Africa, who proposed that this was a protective emotion rather than a physiological state. Some of the signals the "governor" uses to adjust your output include the mix of O_2 and CO_2 in your bloodstream and lactate levels within muscles. These adjustments occur outside of your control—for the most part. There are, however, two ways to manipulate them in your favor. First, there's the hard route, which is just to push yourself harder and tolerate the discomfort. Then there's the easy route: working out your primary breathing muscles, just as you do with any other muscles in order to make them stronger. When you strengthen your breathing muscles, you decrease the level of fatigue felt by the muscles in your arms and legs. This in turn decreases the fatigue signals being sent back to your brain, and encourages the "governor" to let you keep going.

HOW DO YOU RECOVER BETWEEN SETS?

You recover between sprints or sets, and also from day to day. In the first case it is about catching your breath: in the second it is about your body healing (and growing) from the workout. Seven pointers to keep in mind during your workout:

1. Breathe horizontally.
2. During hard efforts, use both nasal and buccal breathing (nose and mouth).
3. Look out into the distance.
4. Note that moment where you go from slightly panicked to "I'm going to be OK." Give that place a name (color or number) that resonates with you.
5. Rather than continuing to try to slow your breath, take two more huge breaths.
6. Pause on exhale, lengthen each exhale.
7. Switch to your nose, flare your nostrils, and relax your jaw.

YOUR STORY

"As a CrossFitter, the time between sets is precious. I counted how many breaths it usually takes me to recover. I forced myself to redefine a good breath as a horizontal one. And now that I know, anatomically, that that big heaving shoulder breath just keeps my heart rate up and needs more breaths to satisfy me. It's been a game changer."

—*Michael A.*

FREQUENTLY ASKED QUESTIONS

Q: **You mention that some athletes have Inspiratory Muscle Training (IMT). What do they do?**

A: *Anything that makes it harder to breathe is theoretically an inspiratory muscle trainer, whether it involves breathing through one nostril or both nostrils, a straw, or through a specific mouthpiece or mask that limits how much air you can pull in. However, listen up, this is important: Unless you correct your biomechanics, breathing any of these will automatically make things worse! You'll be training the wrong muscles and actually encouraging a bad style of breathing. One reason I recommend the O2 Trainer is because I first evaluated the breathing of the founder, Bas Rutten. He has an A+ B-IQ breath and understands and explains the importance of a lower-body breath.*

Q: **What about Expiratory Muscle Training?**

A: *EMT has gotten far less attention because we assume everyone exhales as a "recoil." So, if you are breathing vertically, your exhale is going to be terrible. A recoiling exhale is one of the reasons we have so much misdiagnosed and undertreated asthma and COPD. To work on your exhale, make sure you get Exhale Pulsations and balloon work into your regimen. Especially if you have an average or somewhat heavier body type.*

EXERCISES

BELLOWS BREATH

Bellows Breath comes from yoga, and it actually mimics the high-volume breathing you do when you are going hard. First: inhale as wide as you can, then exhale to as narrow as you can. Unlike Exhale Pulsations you can move your body as you do these. Now speed it up without losing the width of your inhale or contraction of your exhale.

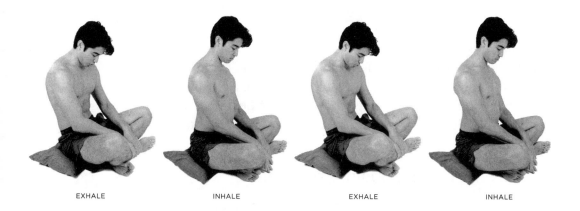

EXHALE   INHALE   EXHALE   INHALE

BEGINNERS LEVEL

15 seconds of Bellows Breath
Inhale once then slowly exhale for 15 seconds
2 consecutive sets
Time: 1 minute

INTERMEDIATE LEVEL

25 seconds of Bellows Breath
Inhale once then slowly exhale for 25 seconds
2-4 consecutive sets

ADVANCED LEVEL

45 seconds of Bellows Breath
Inhale once then slowly exhale for 45 seconds
1-5 consecutive sets
Minimum time: 90 seconds

ASK YOURSELF

What is your max? How long can you go without sacrificing quality? When you fatigue should give you some very solid feedback about how strong your breathing muscles are.

TROUBLESHOOT

If this feels easy, you are doing it wrong. Each inhale has to be wide and the exhale narrow. Remind yourself: you are trying to work out the muscles, so, sure, you could just do half a breath in and out, but this defeats the purpose. You should be hearing both the inhale and exhale loudly; you are a bellows. The tendency is to slack on the inhale.

INHALE MUSCLE TRAINING

O2 Trainer—an inspiratory muscle trainer that limits the amount of air you pull in.[2]

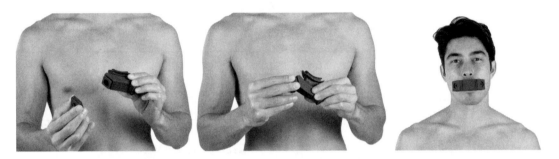

1.   See which mouthpiece hole feels right for you. Then take the one that is slightly bigger (easier). Have someone measure you so that your inhale is the number of the inhales that you took the last time you measured your middle.

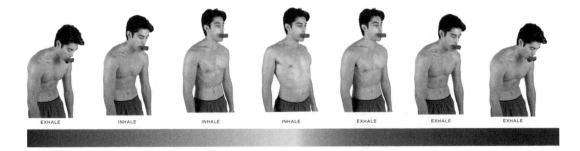

EXHALE   INHALE   INHALE   INHALE   EXHALE   EXHALE   EXHALE

---

2   If you want to know the numbers on how much that is, you can consider the POWERbreathe K series for a baseline assessment.

2. Write down how many breaths before you hit your max (meaning before your inhale and exhale numbers deteriorate). This is your baseline and the number from which you should work up.

ALL WRONG

Watch someone untrained use the O2. They will pick a hard setting, breathe with their upper chest, and their breath will get more and more dominated by auxiliary muscles.

DO THIS NOW

Super-advanced exercises are going into a side plank and doing Bellows Breath for time, or adding the O2 Trainer to side plank breathing.[3]

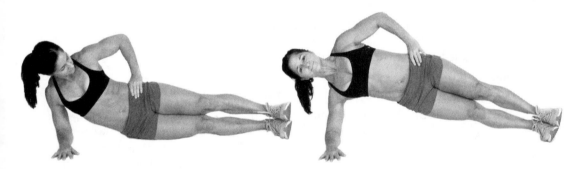

---

3   Stu McGill is our go-to for all things plank: www.backfitpro.com.

WARMING UP YOUR DIAPHRAGM

Dr. Leiter does a set of twenty-five Bellows Breaths before starting a run. "While we don't have the data yet, I am seeing that you start already feeling 'warmed up' rather than waiting to kick into that feeling of being in sync with your body."[4]

EXHALE MUSCLE TRAINING

Your inhale is only as good as your exhale. Few, if any, breathing muscle trainings focus on the exhale, but we do.

> "Exercise performance is partially limited by the functionality of the respiratory musculature. Training these muscles improves steady-state exercise performance. Our data indicate RMW (Respiratory Muscle Warm-up) may enhance short-term, high-intensity exercise performance, but only when performed at an optimal intensity (i.e., airflow restriction). Identifying 'optimal inspiration intensity' (which differs from person to person) is the key."[5]

EXERCISES FOR EXTENDED EXHALE

1. Make your breath a steady stream of air, and time it.
2. Start at ten seconds.
3. Keep adding five seconds each time, with the goal of getting to sixty seconds.

> Joe Rogan's Float Tank Breath is one that he describes as inhaling for 30 seconds and extending the exhale 30 seconds on his podcast, *The Joe Rogan Experience*, episode #460 (with BJJ legend Kron Gracie, who explains the importance of training the diaphragm "like a push-up" and how the breath gets you into an "animal-like state").

---

4   Personal correspondence, May 14, 2018.

5   "Effects of Respiratory Muscle Warm-up on High-Intensity Exercise Performance." An expert at how to balance health in a digital world, Dr. Andy Galpin is a professor at the Center for Sport Performance at California State University, Fullerton, and coauthor of *Unplugged: Evolve from Technology to Upgrade Your Fitness, Performance and Consciousness*. Galpin is gifted at making scientific concepts palatable (and both interesting and actionable).

EXHALE PULSATIONS

Exhale Pulsations are short, sharp exhales where you don't move your back. The inhale is passive. The average for an athlete is 120 pulsations in a row, but the more you can do, the better. You can do these through your nose or mouth.

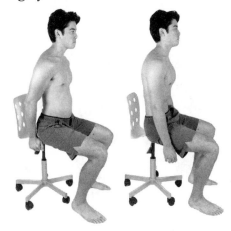

Below are two variations of exercises that utilize Exhale Pulsations.

DOWNWARD DOG

DROP, PICK IT UP

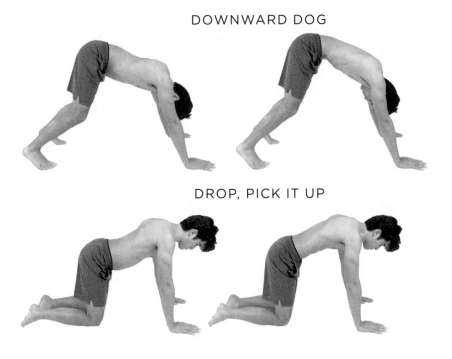

BALLOONS

Your common household balloon is the best EMT device there is. So take the biggest inhale you can, and then exhale using only the middle of your body. You can do one balloon at a time, and move to having two, one in each hand, when you want to move up to an advanced exercise.

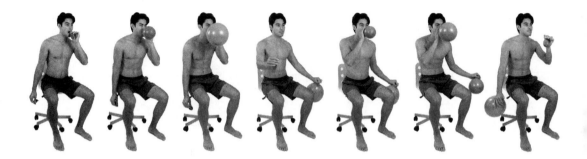

TROUBLESHOOT

1. Keep your face, neck, and shoulders relaxed.
2. If you find you are getting light-headed, realize that much of it has to do with unnecessary pressure in your face. Make sure this feels like an ab exercise.
3. Catch yourself going from a real squeeze (hollowing out) to just a brace. The former is a good exhale, and latter (just bracing down) is not. But if it is what you were used to, you will default to it if you let down your guard.

Challenge yourself: You want the most balloons with the least amount of time. So, you have to take a big breath, then really exhale hard, and you have to do it fast.

TWO QUESTIONS TO ASK YOURSELF BEFORE GOING TO THE NEXT CHAPTER

With all the endurance sports we are discussing, a mechanically sound circumferential/horizontal breath (whether that be lateral or a "back breath") that does not use auxiliary muscles as primary breathing muscles is going to be the more energy-efficient breath. It is a larger breath by definition so that you have more flexibility in your rhythm. Whether you are running, biking, rowing, or swimming, in endurance sports your rate of movement is affected by—if not dictated by—your breath. So, those two questions to ask yourself are:

1. *Am I taking the biggest breath possible?* Keep in mind that an inefficient upper-body breath means you have to take several shallow breaths to make up for one efficient one. And you have to switch to a faster breathing pattern when you are tired, which means you are in the red and the end is near.

2. *Are the ten pounds of breathing muscles that I have strong?* How do I push that wall back so that I have better endurance? The answer is right here: make sure you are using the biggest part of your lungs (LOM), and make sure your breathing muscles are trained and powerful just like any other muscle in your body.

10

SEA, LAND, AND AIR(DYNE): APPLIED TECHNIQUES FOR ROWING, SWIMMING, AND BIKING

ROWING: THREE DIFFERENT BEASTS—OPEN, FLAT, AND LAND

OPEN

Imagine yourself in the middle of the Atlantic. You've been rowing for fifty days and grabbed only eighty-five minutes of uninterrupted sleep. Suddenly your oar fails to strike the water. Mathew Bennett, captain of Team Essence,[1] told me that this "miss of the water that occurs with ocean rowing is as jarring as the recoil from a blow that does not connect in boxing. I'd hear a team member grunt or yell and know the angle of the boat had caused him to miss water, and end up striking himself in the face or chest. When this happens, your brain scrambles to get your balance back—and then you try to focus on your breathing. In this case, the focus on breathing is more for stabilization."[2]

FLAT

Flat water rowing uses vivid dramatic descriptors: the boat is an entity that breathes, and the rowers cumulatively are its inhale and exhale. Rowing and breathing in unison, consequently, is criti-

---

1   In 2016 Team Essence rowed across the Atlantic *unsupported*, with a time of 50 days, 10 hours, 36 minutes (Portugal to Venezuela).

2   Interview, December 10, 2018.

cal. Every breath, every stroke, the rower connects. Two-time Olympic medalist and coach Erin Cafaro likens it to military marching, where the energy of the pace and breath connect: "Even what seems like a minor detail, like having someone sitting behind you on the boat who is breathing out of sync, is easily perceptible, and contagious." The profound motivation and synchronized energy the group dynamic creates is evident once the boat crosses the finish line: the rowers collapse and allow themselves to default to erratic gasping for air in order to recover.[3]

"With rowing, you have to combine the explosive power of a linebacker on the drive with the savviness of a ninja on the recovery. You can't have tension, even in your feet, on the recovery or you'll slow down the boat. One of my favorite coaching cues is, 'let the boat breathe.' The boat moves the most on the recovery phase of the stroke if you allow it. 'Free speed' happens when you let it go; when you have the patience and skill to let the boat run off of the good effort you just put in on the drive. It's what differentiates a good boat from a great boat," Cafaro points out.

LAND

The traditional recommendation for breathing on the indoor rowing machine (also known as the "erg") is as follows:

"Battle paddle" is when the person rowing next to you has a similar rhythm and speed and you race each other in a competitive or collegial spirit.

1. During low-intensity rowing (one breath): Exhale on the drive, expelling all remaining air at the finish; inhale on the recovery up to the catch.
2. During high-intensity rowing (two breaths): Exhale on the drive and catch. Small inhales will happen naturally between the two.

DO THIS NOW

Use rowing to measure your endurance. Keeping all the other metrics the same, see exactly at what stroke rate or effort level you switch from one breath to two. As you change your

---

3   Personal correspondence, November 12, 2018.

breath to a horizontal one and strengthen your breathing muscles, you will see alterations over the next few days and weeks. Make sure you are diligent about writing your baseline numbers, and keep track as they change.

Some specific points to stress are:

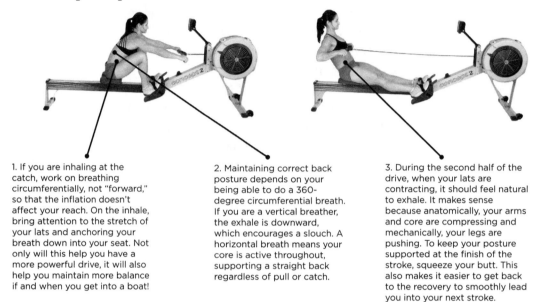

1. If you are inhaling at the catch, work on breathing circumferentially, not "forward," so that the inflation doesn't affect your reach. On the inhale, bring attention to the stretch of your lats and anchoring your breath down into your seat. Not only will this help you have a more powerful drive, it will also help you maintain more balance if and when you get into a boat!

2. Maintaining correct back posture depends on your being able to do a 360-degree circumferential breath. If you are a vertical breather, the exhale is downward, which encourages a slouch. A horizontal breath means your core is active throughout, supporting a straight back regardless of pull or catch.

3. During the second half of the drive, when your lats are contracting, it should feel natural to exhale. It makes sense because anatomically, your arms and core are compressing and mechanically, your legs are pushing. To keep your posture supported at the finish of the stroke, squeeze your butt. This also makes it easier to get back to the recovery to smoothly lead you into your next stroke.

ROWING INSTRUCTIONS

1. Grab the handle with both hands and put your arms straight out in front of you.
2. Push your legs and seat back at the same time while hanging on the handle with straight arms.
3. Once your legs are almost flat, lean back and thrust your hips open and bring your arms and the handle in with your elbows down by your sides at a 90-degree angle.
4. Push your arms out straight around belly button level.
5. Pivot forward from the hips, until your shoulders are slightly in front of your hips.
6. Release your knees and allow your seat to come back up the slide. You should arrive in the same position in which you started.

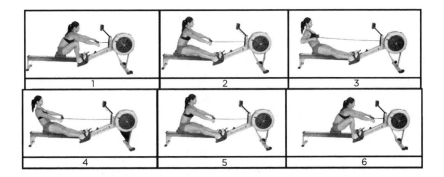

BREATHING INSTRUCTIONS

1. Inhale, feeling your back and sides expand at the catch.
2. Exhale with a leg push on the drive (part one).
3. Continue to exhale as arms draw to body to the finish (part two).
4. Inhale to start the recovery with arms away.
5. Continue to inhale on the recovery (if high intensity, add another breath revolution).
6. Inhale at the catch, feeling your sides and back expand.

NOTE

Once you have learned to feel your breathing expand at your sides and even your back, your breath should not affect your reach. Notice when you need to switch to mouth breathing and when you need two breaths a stroke. This should be a metric that you use to get better.

TROUBLESHOOT

The breath is not directly correlated with the catch or the finish positions. Notice if your inhale continues around the catch as you start to push on the drive. Or if you need to take an additional inhale and exhale as you start to come up the slide on the recovery. As your stroke rate and intensity increases, your breathing will become more fluid and might not match up exactly with the catch or finish.

FREQUENTLY ASKED QUESTIONS

Q: Isn't the exhale supposed to be relaxing?

A: *Yes, if you are paddling on a serene lake with your lover and a picnic basket. If you are battle paddling in the gym, absolutely not. Your inhale is aggressive and your exhale is aggressive.*

NOTE: PUTTING ON THE BRAKES

What do you do with the breath as you switch movements when changing direction of the catch or pull? Some movements are "harmonic," and involve a pendulum-like cadence. Others (e.g., free running or parkour) need more of a break and require you to use the exhale as an internal shock absorption. With downhill skiing, there might be an exhale at the apex of a sharp curve, and you might even hear yourself grunt. A different type of challenge is the sharp movements you can't predict, as in mountain or trail biking, when your breath and core have to control both your body and the bike's momentum.

> *While anatomically the exhale is more "relaxing" in that the heart rate slows slightly, the fact is that the body needs to soften and relax to get a really good inhale.*

CATCH-22

When you switch to a faster breath—in running, swimming, biking, or rowing—that increase will absorb energy. If it is not an efficient breath (cf. B-IQ), then it will be using more energy than it produces. A faster breath feels good initially, but then it "loses" that sensation of fueling you and you are winded again. The goal is to make your breath efficient and train your breathing muscles to use *primary* breathing muscles instead of *auxiliary* ones. Keep in mind that stronger breathing muscles require *less oxygen*. You can stay at a slower breath rate longer, and when you switch you'll be able to feel fueled longer as well. It's the sensation of having more "gas." The extensive research on inspiratory muscle training explains all this in very technical terms, but we've broken it down, and added expiratory muscle training to the recommendations as well.

YOUR STORIES

"I went abroad for two weeks and did breathing exercises religiously in hopes of not 'losing' all my conditioning. It worked, and when I got back on the rower at home, I stopped and changed rowers because I thought the rower might not have been correctly calibrated!"

—*Mattie L.*

Once you have an "A" B-IQ, mosey on over to www.shiftstate.io for the breathing app I love.

"I use rowing as part of interval training, on an erg for the standard of 500–2000 meters while keeping track of wattage and time. For me the inhales are really gulps of air, not full breaths. The exhales are more thorough and perceptible."

—*Jennifer T.*

"After trying breathing in all different ways, I found that focusing on 'the count' worked best for me. Two counts for the catch, one count out as I push with my legs (calling this 'the pull' adds to the confusion), so that my inhale was slower than my exhale."

—*Phillip M.*

"When doing interval training, the first time I sit down at the rower I know that I can keep a one-breath-per-stroke movement, but the second time around, I know I am tired and that I should start with a two-breath inhale/exhale tempo so as not to lose speed. You are pushing yourself on both on the inhale and exhale. The exhale is a moment to get back to the inhale; it's not really a recovery. When you are going fast, the exhale is a contraction to help you get back to the inhale."

—*Cody S.*

"I used to only be able to stay at one breath per stroke the first minute. As my breathing muscles have gotten stronger I've been steadily gaining seconds before having to shift into two breaths a stroke."

—*Alicia B.*

THE ART OF BREATH GEARS

G1
Working Cadence 1a
- Equal: Nasal In/Nasal Out
> *Low Aerobic*

G2
Working SuperVentilation 1
- Power Nasal In/Nasal Out
> *High Aerobic*

G3
Working Bellows Breath
- Power Nasal In/Power Nasal Out
> *Anaerobic Threshold (Transition)*

G4
Working SuperVentilation 2
- Nasal In/Mouth Out
> *Low Anaerobic*

G5
Working SuperVentilation 3
- Mouth In/Mouth Out
> *High Anaerobic*

THE ART OF BREATH CALLS IT "USING YOUR GEARS"

Breathing only through the nose allows you to work at a low to moderate pace. It's perfect for developing an aerobic base, which makes it great for activities like running, rowing, and cycling. As your efforts become more intense (and more anaerobic), you begin to incorporate the mouth more. "By learning these gears, you are actually learning exactly how to understand and manage intensity," explains Brian Mackenzie, founder of The Art of Breath Program.[5] The concept of gears is nothing short of brilliant because it brings body awareness to something traditionally left to chance.

> The more efficient your breath is, the longer you can go in your sequence. Ask yourself, how can I be more intentional in my short breath holds, in my release of breath. This will lead to a more perfect marriage of tension and fluidity. Breathing is an "internal movement" where you have to be especially aware. When you become one with your kettlebell, the breath allows you to be more ballistic and achieve flow, your isometric holds turn into dynamic movement and you really grasp fluidity.[4]
>
> — Marcus Martinez, kettlebell expert

---

4   Interview with Marcus Martinez, founder of Living.Fit, on March 30, 2019.

5   Interview with Brian MacKenzie on February 2, 2019.

THE OPPOSITE ADVICE: TRADITIONAL OR REVERSE BREATH IN ROWING?

When you row, do you inhale as push on the drive? Or do you exhale?

Traditionally, rowing encourages an inhale at the catch and an exhale on the drive. But there are some that make the argument you should do the opposite: exhale at the catch and inhale on the drive. The Reverse Breath is also favored by some kettlebell experts who encourage an inhale on the "up" phase of the swing for better endurance.

Xeno Müller, an Olympic gold and silver medalist and coach at Elite Rowing Coach, is in the Reverse Breath camp. "Absolute relaxation occurs through exhaling. . . . As the acceleration progresses and the upper body swings open the lungs fill with air and provide a strong finish position."[6]

Marc Monplaisir, competitive master sculler at the Ever Green Boat Club in New Jersey agrees. He backed up Xeno by adding "being fully inflated" at the point of maximum compression means that you are losing an inch or two of stroke length. . . . [Exhaling] allows you to be fully relaxed and extended at the catch, giving you room to get a couple more inches of length."[7]

Erin Cafaro, a two-time Olympic gold medalist, defends the traditional breath: "Our maximum load and power potential is at the catch. Using a low diaphragmatic inhale coming into the catch will allow our core muscles to create a 'weight belt' to support our precious spine and nervous system and signal all systems are a-go to push hard on the drive. More compression or length at the catch is not a good excuse to sacrifice the sanctity of our spine and potential power output."[8]

> Mountaineers will go so far as to teach people to breathe in through their nose and mouth simultaneously, while also flaring the nostrils. Your tongue is the lever that makes your breath either completely nasal or oral. Leaving your tongue neutral and mouth open results in an oralbuccal breath. In a pinch you can get air in and out through both orifices.

---

6   https://www.row2k.com/blogs/post/2/49/Rowing-is-not-weight-lifting--breathe-accordingly-/.

7   https://crossfitrowingblog.com/2015/04/24/breathing-technique-for-rowing/?wref=tp.

8   Personal correspondence, November 12, 2018.

DO THIS NOW: ROWING BREATH REVERSALS

1. Do 20 breaths traditional.
2. Do 20 reverse-row breaths.
3. Take a break, then do it again, this time starting with the reverse-row breath first.

Which felt more natural? Most importantly, which felt more supportive to your spine? Then, more nuanced questions follow: How did switching the breath affect your form, time, and output? What movements are similar and how do we breathe in those? Is it useful to be able to do the movement with both styles of breathing for flexibility of rhythm?

With some movements the division is clear: Some are mechanical, others are clearly ana- tomical; others start as anatomical and as they get harder, switch to mechanical.

Rowing has more of an integrative breath than other endurance sports, such as running, due to the deliberate power and recovery phase and the lower cadence. The rowing stroke is both a fluid and power-producing movement that allows for both the bracing of the mechanical breath and the continuity of the anatomical breath.

> How long can you stay in a 1:1 breath? How long can you stay breathing nasally? Be the exper- imenter and see what is habit, what makes sense intellectually, and how you can challenge yourself in a new way.

Whether you like to inhale at the catch or at the finish of the stroke, the most important part to remember while rowing is to be conscious of the bracing and the rhythm of your breathing. For now, just make sure you notice which one you are using. Do not default to a breathing style that does not support your spine when necessary, or to holding your breath when you shouldn't.

SWIMMING

Swimming is a compelling example of how the breath affects movement—rather than tagging along or just ignoring it alto- gether. The efficiency and control of your breath when swimming is paramount because they dictate success. Swimming is breathing with movement attached. You can't muscle through it. Breathe haphazardly when swimming owing to lack of thoughtfulness and you will find yourself in a panic and nowhere near the side of the pool or near land.

If you have taken up swimming as an adult or come back to it as a result of injury because it is a "safe" sport, you'll soon realize that becoming proficient is more about controlling your breath than co-ordinating or strengthening your arms and legs. Keep in mind that:

1. Rib cage flexibility should be the main focus in your breathing training because the size of the inhale depends on the expansion of the sides of your ribs.

2. You are never completely inhaled or exhaled; you are "grabbing a bite" of air. You have to be able to get used to this feeling.

3. Your inhale has to be fast; your exhale has to be controlled. Both depend on the strength and coordination of your breathing muscles. For the inhale, your diaphragm has to be strong (in order to pull air in fast); for the exhale, your internal intercostals and obliques have to be strong (in order to control the push of the exhale).

HOW TO "GRAB A BITE" OF AIR

1. Breathe at the corner of the mouth. Don't "over roll" in order to get your mouth completely out of the water. Just "grab a bite" of air with the corner of your mouth. Exhale on the side, not when your face is directly down.

2. Breathing when doing the crawl is the opposite of breathing on land in that you inhale through the mouth and exhale through the nose. It's one of the reasons that for a newbie swimmer it can feel awkward in the beginning.

3. Swimming doesn't have the luxury of a consistently satisfying complete inhale or exhale. In fact, there may be an overlap between both. (Much like the circular breathing of the Australian wind instrument, the didgeridoo.)

MERMAIDS, UNDERWATER DANCES, AND AMMO CARRIES

In 1946, Newton Perry, a former U.S. Navy sailor who trained SEALs to swim underwater in World War II, visited Weeki Wachee, Florida, and decided to open a small mermaid school there. Fast-forward to August 2012: the Mermaid Kat Academy, made "mermaiding" accessible to everyone. Shortly after that, the Philippine Mermaid Swimming Academy and several other mermaid schools opened around the world. Think it's easy to be a mermaid? Try eating a banana and smiling underwater in a fifteen-pound mermaid suit with your feet bound by your heavy prosthetic tail. Pool workouts are big lately, and folks usually think of ammo carries, but mermaiding is tough. And these beauties are hard-core when it comes to breath holding.

Stew Smith, a graduate of the US Naval Academy, a former Navy SEAL Lieutenant, and author of several fitness and self-defense books, is one of the most sought-after experts on Spec Ops Level workouts, especially pool workouts. Here's his step-by-step guide to "grabbing a bite of air":

1. The biggest mistake I see is overworking: a lot of kicking and using big muscle groups that suck up all your oxygen.

2. Then it's poor technique: you see folks who don't exhale underwater, then they don't have enough time to exhale and inhale when they come up. All you should be doing when your head comes up is inhaling.

3. I always say, don't be a seesaw, be a screwdriver, meaning you should turn to breathe during the stroke, not pop up. If you pop up your feet will drop and then you'll just be treading water.[9]

> Laird Hamilton and Gabrielle Reece's brainchild, XPT, has popularized pool workouts, which add an undeniable buzz to an otherwise bland routine in gym workouts. My favorite in the pool are jump squats, which can be done in shallow water without weight, with a weight in each hand in a deeper part of the pool, or with a kettlebell.

If you are feeling rushed, it's because you are not timing your exhale and it's bleeding into your inhale time. Timing and using your tongue to be the gatekeeper between the inhale and exhale is part of the practice. Janet Evans, three-time Olympian and four-time individual Olympic gold medalist, and author of *Total Swimming*, describes submerging her head and body underwater repeatedly, blowing the air out of her nose, emptying her lungs via bubbling before she surfaced to help internalize this process. If you would rather start by blowing through a straw into a glass of water before getting into the pool, keep it from spraying and keep it continuous. She recounts, "Learning to exhale in a slow controlled way was excruciating but addictive. It wasn't about holding my breath at all; it was way harder actually. I had to control the bubbles so they were a steady stream."

---

9   Interview, December 10, 2018. Watch his precision get better after an hour in freezing water: http://www.stewsmith.com/linkpages/hypothermia.htm.

DO THIS NOW

Work your exhale muscles by doing fast movements (e.g., Exhale Pulsations) and by timing and extending your continuous exhale. Can you exhale a steady stream of air for thirty seconds? Forty-five? Sixty? How is your timing, meaning when you get to your desired number do you have more air left, or the opposite—are you holding your breath because you don't have enough? In a sport like swimming, these seemingly fine details make the difference between an advanced breather and a superior one.

YOUR STORY

"I went back to swimming because I was injured and my PT recommended it. Initially it felt like such a struggle it was exhausting. Once I broke it down and understood that my breathing was affecting my buoyancy and pace, it all fell into place and I wasn't flailing and trying to muscle through it the way I do things on land."

—*Liam C.*

BIKING

The critical connection between oxygen and energy has been extensively studied among cyclists. In effect, it is one of the first sports to include inspiratory muscle workouts in their training.

Mechanically, for a cyclist, efficient breathing requires mostly a lateral and back breath because the front body is also being used for stabilization in a bent-over posture. As with rowing, the type of biking you are doing has a major influence on your breathing: whether the course is on a trail or highway, whether it's competitive cyclist-to-cyclist, against the clock, or you are more balanced as on an assault bike or in a spin class.

DO THIS NOW

Right now, hop on a stationary bike and consider these three topics:

1. As compared to rowing, there is no "rest" time. Learning to pace yourself is critical because it may not be built into the movement.
2. Notice which is your kick leg—it's the one that "keeps time." Even when going hard, there is one foot that is more "dominant" than the other. To counter this, you should "switch the kick"; that is to say, switch your attention to the less dominant leg when you feel fatigue or are losing focus.
3. Notice how you brace less on a stationary bike, and hence a lower-body breath is possible. On roads or trails, bracing of the body and bike means an expansive abdominothoracic breath is not realistic. Working on the expansion of your sides and back means you will continue to breathe efficiently, which will make a noticeable difference in your energy level.

EXERCISE

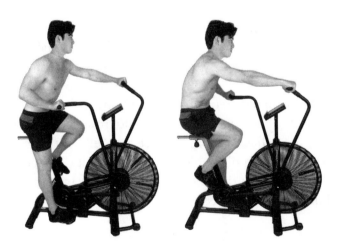

ASSAULT BIKE

Let's say that your kick leg is your right leg. Move it to your left (meaning switch your attention to your left and lean on it more). Now focus on your right arm, then on your left. Finally make the opposing arm and leg your "kick." Your exhale and the "kick" are connected. Being able to breathe in different situations and postures makes you own the sport more. In addition, the cross-body movements are a good brain exercise.

STAIRS—RUNNING TO A HARD PACE

Firefighter Jimmy Lopez, founder, owner, and operator of Monkey Bar Gymnasium in New York, has climbed millions of stairs over the years. In an interview he told me: "We don't run up the stairs with our gear. Our job begins once we actually reach the fire floor. Burning yourself out on the stairs is counterproductive and could disrupt your performance for the rest of the fire. You have to pace yourself so that when you get there you can work. I make sure that I am not exclusively breathing from my mouth. Much like running to a hard pace. I mix in some nasal inhales to act as a governor to my pace. I make sure I am exhaling well, and I will forcefully exhale after so many breaths. Also I use everything to help me based on tools I am carrying. If I can grab a railing to help pull or if I have a hook, I use it like a trekking pole."

ENDURANCE AND EMERGENCY AIR MANAGEMENT

Until now, breath training for firefighters focused on the time spent in "masking up" and on instructions on how to remain calm and conserve oxygen. The pointers were few; e.g., use Skip Breathing, which means holding your breath intermittently between respirations, or Reilly Breathing, which includes a hum on the exhale with the goal of helping conserve the oxygen tank.

The greatest threat firefighters encounter is when the low-air alarm sounds, and they find themselves in a pitch-black room, searching to find a way out, or becoming panicked in a confined space. They are very aware that smoke inhalation means lung damage or even death. Given the rise of rural fires, there is a substantial amount of research being conducted that examines the effect of exhaustion and the skills and resources needed when large-scale, long-duration natural disasters occur.

One challenge that these first responders face is not just carrying heavy gear, but gear that weighs more on one side (e.g., rope) and consequently requires more bracing. The mask restricts breathing to an extent that an inhale is a "pull in" of air that requires more breathing muscle involvement.

While spirometry remains the standard tool that determines lung damage, therapies to restore lung volume and speed as measured by spirometry are still not well integrated into respiratory physiology. Programs such as the FDNY's MPI (Mental Performance Initiative) are cutting edge in their incorporation of breathing training due to their endurance and active-recovery curriculum. Newest discussions center around endurance and resilience (about which we'll talk more later).

Correcting the location of breathing and the strengthening of breathing muscles can impact the performance of firefighters and first responders in the following ways:

1. Heart rate can be better managed.
2. Panic can be controlled; consequently, auditory skills and memory can be controlled.
3. Endurance apart from cardio can be enhanced.
4. Awareness that the diaphragm is both a breathing muscle and a muscle of balance, crucial when carrying load, can be heightened.
5. Experiencing discomfort can be practiced, especially when the mask air restriction is uncomfortable, which in turn affects the CO_2-O_2 balance.
6. Breathing for active recovery from day to day, which clearly aids in detoxification of the body, can be incorporated into training.
7. Breathing exercises and breath-led meditation are a big part of mental performance and resilience training for first responders.

FREQUENTLY ASKED QUESTIONS

Q: **My tennis instructor told me to make my exhale audible, sort of like a loud hum. What's that about?**

A: *That is a simple technique used in several sports to make sure you don't hold your breath when hitting.*

CONCLUSION

Regardless of your sport, you should include some component of a high-intensity workout in your practice. A summary of breathing exercises for endurance sports is as follows:

1. Every movement has a breath that is attached to it, be it anatomical (when your spine extends as you inhale and vice versa) or mechanical (you brace to protect your spine or exhale with effort—but more of that in the next chapter).
2. Recovery between exercises has to be deliberate. Breathe horizontally to get rid of lactic acid and make up your oxygen debt, and you will recover sooner between sets and from one day to the next.
3. Exercise your breathing muscles apart from your sport. This will improve your endurance. Science has proved it; now we have the practical application to follow.

11

BREATHING FOR STRENGTH: DISCOVER YOUR INNER ANACONDA

HISTORY: "QUIET BREATHING IS AN ABOMINATION"

You would think that breathing while lifting would be second nature to all of us. Both lifting and carrying rank among the top activities in which humans—and our hominid ancestors—have engaged. Archaeological research reports that Neanderthals would carry fifty-plus-pound hunks of meat for up to thirty miles. And then repeat the slog for up to two weeks after killing a woolly mammoth. Stone Age peoples in Libya moved ninety-pound blocks with the help of cattle, but even with the beasts of burden bearing the brunt of the work, someone had to chuck the weight onto their backs.

The use of "explosive strength" became a necessity when people started hurling spears at prey—around 90,000 years ago. Life didn't get that much easier when humans transitioned to farming. A farmer working in the Fertile Crescent during the early days of agriculture (around 12,000 years ago) had to clear entire fields of grain by sickle. Hello, rotational strength. And that is to say nothing of all the plowing, the planting, the lifting, and carrying needed to collect and bag the wheat, barley, millet, and emmer into shacks for drying, then carting to the granaries for storage, and finally onto boats for shipping down the Euphrates or Tigris.

About 3,000 years ago, humans started using their muscles in a different way: hitting the gym. The earliest recorded gymnasiums (literally in Greek, "places to train naked") date back that far. If you were to step into the Academy or the Lyceum, the two most famous gyms in Athens, you'd have seen large open-air spaces where men (and they were places exclusively for men) ran, threw javelins and discs, and wrestled.

With the fall of the Greco-Roman empire, gymnasiums disappeared—and stayed obscured throughout the Dark Ages. Fitness as such didn't return as a public pursuit until 1811, when a Prussian patriot named Friedrich Jahn, who was still smarting over his country's loss to Napoleon five years prior, launched a Turnplatz, or "exercise field," outside Berlin. In fact, Jahn invented gear like the parallel bars and other equipment that formed the basis for gymnastics.

Many cite the late 1800s and early 1900s as the birth of the concept of fitness as we know it today. During that time, the first commercial gyms sprang up in France and England. One gym founded by Eugen Sandow in England in many ways resembled what you see today in your neighborhood, with personal trainers leading people through prescribed weight-training workouts.

As gyms spread, so did debates over how one should go about breathing while training. Sandow, for example, advised all trainees to breathe in through the nose and out through the mouth. So did strength pioneer George Hackenschmidt, who also happens to be the man who gave the "Hack Squat" its name. Bernarr Macfadden, a bodybuilding buff and publisher akin to Joe Weider (but who lived three decades before Weider published issue number one of *Your Physique*) who was a fan of audible breathing and grunts, said "quiet breathing [was] used by weaklings," and called it an abomination. (More on groaning and grunting at the gym coming up.)

One of the biggest societal concerns of Sandow's[1] era was industrialization. Sandow even titled a book *Life Is Movement*, and posited that by limiting how much people moved, modern living was making people sickly and overweight. If industrialization was bad for people's health, then what we have today—technologization—might be even worse. Today's sedentary and computer-centric culture has all but eliminated physical activity from nine to five. For

---

1   Interesting to note, Sandow was an avid yogi and an expert on military readiness. Ahead of his time, he believed that exercise could help with depression.

most, any of the lifting, carrying, and other grunt-necessitating work we do takes place at the gym, which is a big reason why fitness has become big business. Today, about one out of every five Americans has a gym membership; most work out there about an hour three times per week while trying to undo the damage from all of the sitting they do during the other fifteen or so waking hours during the day.[2]

THE STRENGTH EXPERTS WEIGH IN

A fundamental shift has been taking place in strength training due to the fact that, until a few years ago, many mainstream strength coaches ignored breathing. Even great ones. Mike Boyle of Mike Boyle Strength and Conditioning in Boston, for example, is regarded by many as a premier performance coach and thought leader in the industry. When Boyle speaks, in-the-know coaches listen. And in 2008, while discussing breathing in a post on his blog, Boyle wrote, "Please stop telling me about the breathing. I can't tell you how many times people have told me that my athletes really don't know how to breathe and that yoga will totally change them. Thank God I have never had an athlete stop breathing on me." However, six years later, Boyle completely changed course, saying: "Now I would tell you that every good coach that I know is incorporating some type of breathing exercise into their routines . . . it's a topic we kinda missed the boat on. I know I personally missed the boat. I have some articles coming out where I apologize to the yoga people I made fun of for talking about breathing exercises."

> "Breathing is a fundamental athletic skill—like a squat—and it should be taught."
>
> —Pavel Tsatsouline, *The Naked Warrior*

Strength and conditioning coach Joe DeFranco, owner of De-Franco's Gym, voted one of America's 10 Best Gyms by *Men's Health* magazine, stated, "There are just so many benefits [to training breathing] . . . It can improve your mobility. It improves your posture. It improves endurance. It can help alleviate a ton of pain, we've

---

2   Kufahl, Pamela. "IHRSA Reports 57 Million Health Club Members, $27.6 Billion in Industry Revenue in 2016." *Club Industry,* April 14, 2017.

Sharon Moskowitz, strength and conditioning coordinator of the USA Wheelchair Rugby Team, teaches her athletes to breathe by "filling out" or "seating your body down," which "gives you stability so you can go to higher loads without getting pulled out of the chair." She cues this by focusing on shoulder blade retraction and stacking the shoulders into a stable position.[3]

seen that happen first-hand."[4] Practicing breathing techniques can reduce anxiety, lower oxidative stress, improve the balance of the parasympathetic and sympathetic divisions of the autonomic nervous systems, reduce blood pressure, and reduce resting heart rate.

Specifically, when it comes to strength, breathing poorly can definitely inhibit your lift in quality and weight, and even lead to injury. It causes you to fatigue prematurely, since you are working harder to draw in the oxygen you need (and expel the CO_2 you need to release). In sum, better breathing is the name of the game because it means better movement integrity in strength training. Each breath affects your stability, posture, balance, and range of motion. Proper breathing lowers your center of gravity, which in turn makes you stronger and more mobile. Eric Cressey, founder of Cressey Sports Performance and coach to many MLB players, says, "Once you [correct someone's breathing], what you'll find is that guys get range of motion elsewhere."

The ability to breathe while maintaining tension in your core is necessary for strength training. This is an underappreciated skill, although it's the one that helps you develop full-body strength faster. Better breathing means better bracing and higher 1-rep maxes. Your breath creates intrathoracic and intra-abdominal pressure. This pressure is like a "volume knob" for your strength, according to StrongFirst founder and former Soviet Special Forces soldier Pavel Tsatsouline, who points out that, "The higher this pressure, the greater your strength—and visa versa."

Better breathing also means more energy. Proper breathing mechanics lets you re-oxygenate and keep your O_2/CO_2 balanced. It flushes blood waste products like lactic acid. You'll recover faster between sets and after workouts. And finally, better breathing means greater stability and increased integrity of movement, all of

---

3   Interview on May 18, 2019.

4   Personal communication in October 2018.

which means you will be able to train more consistently and grow stronger.

Breathing wields influence over two things that are critical when it comes to strength: the alignment of your body's structure and the pressure you generate within your body. The two are very much related because your body's posture affects how much internal pressure you can create, which in turn affects the strength you can generate.

ANACONDA STRENGTH: THE BREATHING/ POSTURE CONNECTION

Yes, your breathing and posture are intimately connected. Perhaps the explanation of how your posture affects your body's breathing and strength that's easiest to understand is offered by Mary Massery, DPT, a physical therapist based outside of Chicago. Massery likens the torso to a soda can. And then goes on to clarify that many people are unaware of how strong soda cans are. One could stack more than 1,500 full cans on top of one another before the bottom one supporting all the weight would fail. But it isn't the flimsy aluminum sides that give the cans their fortitude; they get their strength from the pressure contained within. "Pressure creates functional strength to an otherwise weak structure," Massery explains in her delightful YouTube video, "Soda Pop Can Model," adding that the same is true for the body. "The skeleton itself is not strong. It's what holds the skeleton up": the torso, our pressure-containing canister.

"The big thing I'm always looking for is trying to stack the rib cage on top of pelvis. All of my cues are designed for stacking rib cage on top of pelvis," points out Mike Robertson, physical preparation coach and co-owner of

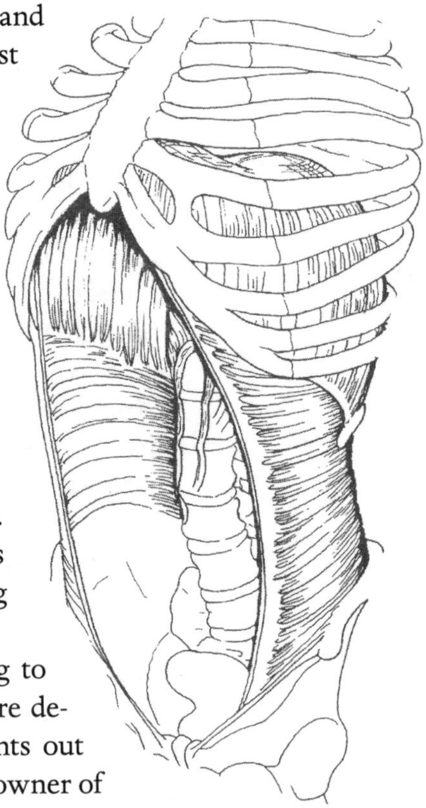

Figure 11.1

IFAST, an elite training center in Indianapolis.[5] However, the problem is that many people aren't in this alignment—or anything close to it. Many people end up in what Robertson describes as "extended posture." Extended posture could look like a recruit standing at attention at Parris Island with a rib cage that's flared outward. Or it could be an anterior pelvic tilt (common in hockey players). Or you could even have both.

Canadian physiotherapist Diane Lee explains in *The Pelvic Girdle* how people will utilize different strategies to transfer loads through the lower back, hips, and pelvis. She calls people who have extended posture "back grippers," because the long muscles in the back (the erector spinae) are working or "gripping" nearly all the time. This posture inhibits expansion of the back of the rib cage during the inhalation phase of breathing. Another posture that inhibits breathing is exhibited by "chest grippers," or people whose ribs seem to be pulled tight into the body.

When your core muscles are performing correctly, your diaphragm and intercostals expand the rib cage circumferentially on an inhale. Meanwhile, at the bottom of the canister, your pelvic floor relaxes. If you were resting and relaxing, your abdomen and rib cage would expand outward slightly. But when you are under load, you brace your middle, and this pressure reinforces the spine and prevents it from buckling, even when it's straining under very heavy loads, according to Dr. Stuart McGill, author of *Low Back Disorders*. Research shows that this creation of intra-abdominal pressure is crucial to keeping your spine safe when you lift. Without it, throwing a bar on your back that stresses your

---

LOUIE SIMMONS EXPLAINS THE VALSALVA MANEUVER

A proper Valsalva comes down to the same two factors that protect you during any lifting technique: "A good breath and a good brace," explains Louie Simmons, powerlifting legend and developer of the Westside Barbell method of training. "Expand your abdomen by taking a deep breath through the diaphragm, pulling as much air as possible into your abdomen."[6] If you are wearing a lifting belt, press your abdominal muscles outward against it. Finish your inhale, then hold your breath and your brace throughout the lowering phase of the lift. You can continue to hold your breath as you push back up, or exhale with a grunt, hiss, or scream as you reach—and push past—the sticking point.

---

5   Personal correspondence, July 15, 2018.
6   Personal correspondence, December 18, 2018.

interspinal muscles (tiny muscles that support the vertebrae) increases the risk of fractures or herniated discs (or both).

Numerous studies document that how you breathe directly impacts intrathoracic and intra-abdominal pressure. This pressure stabilizes the spine and creates core stiffness, which is how you generate strength. "The stiffer your core, the more power transfer across your ball and socket joints—the hips down below, and your shoulders up above," says McGill. Notwithstanding, the act of breathing alone doesn't create this sturdiness; you also need to create an effective brace to contain the pressure. "In order to build up intra-abdominal pressure, you have to turn on your abdominal wall, which adds a squeezing force," adds McGill.[7]

More pressure means heavier lifts, and heavier lifts are the name of the game. "Air is support for the back," says Mark Rippetoe, strength coach and author of *Starting Strength: Basic Barbell Training*. The ability to maintain this brace while performing any activity is the true trick to developing full-body strength. "We call it anaconda strength," says Dan John, strength coach and author of multiple books, including *Now What: The Ongoing Pursuit of Improved Performance*. "Think of a bicycle inner tube. How does it make the tire work? By filling up with pressure."[8] So the trick for any lifter is learning how to effectively create that brace, "fill the tire," and then breathe through it. It sounds simple, but it is more demanding than you think.

> "The cue to 'arch hard' is not the solution. It's not just about the biggest breath or just tensing. You need to contract your body and use your belt as a cue. It's not just 'shoving' everything down into the belt. You are trying to fill all the interior nooks and crannies. Breathing into your lower back and filling up there is one of the toughest cues to understand."[9]
>
> —Jesse Irizarry, owner of JDI Barbell and former competitive powerlifter

---

7   Interview with McGill, July 5, 2018.
8   Interview with John, July 27, 2018.
9   Interview with Irizarry, November 20, 2018.

HOW BRANDON LILLY, TOP-RANKED POWERLIFTER, DEADLIFTS

> *"I walk up to the bar and hold my hands out in front of me. I really try to control my breath and then right before I go taking a series of larger breaths, I think about pushing my rib cage down into my side on top of my belt so I actually have a physical cue. I can feel around my belt and then right before I drop, I draw in one more breath, one more gulp, then I go down and I hold that entire breath through the top. Then at the top I exhale and I let myself go down to the ground pretty quickly. I don't try to have any kind of eccentric resistance; I just kinda let the bar drop to the ground. In training it's a little bit different. I do the series of breaths like before but then I go to one elongated exhale as I lower the bar for a 2 to 3 count."*

THE TOP TEN

To leave you with some food for thought, here are the top ten questions that get asked about breathing and strength training. Some seem self-explanatory, others quirky, but they come up over and over again, so here we go:

Q: **Why do I feel like grunting when I'm working out?**

A: *Here's a story from Belisa: While I was at Gold's Gym in 2006 as part of their advisory board, the topic of grunting came up in the news. I discussed the more unnecessary and attention-seeking guttural groans heard in a "typical after-work workout." That being said, meaningful efficient grunts are good grunts. And there's a good reason for grunting: Research shows that these noises increase your strength. How? When you grunt (or hiss, etc.), you activate your abdominal wall, which increases IAP and core stiffness. "The grunt is very much a performance-enhancing effort," says McGill. So did a 2014 study at Drexel University, in which participants were asked to squeeze a hand dynamometer three different ways: 1) while holding their breath 2) while exhaling, and 3) while exhaling and grunting.*

"[What] we found was that there was actually an additional 10 percent increase in force when yelling," said researcher Chris Rodolico in "The Science of Grunting While Weightlifting," at WHYY.org. So is it better to grunt, or scream, or shout ki-ya! like Bruce Lee? The answer depends on what you're doing. A short, powerful noise like ki-ya! can help you generate a short, powerful strike. "Sudden squeezing of the air by a powerful contraction of the respiratory muscles and the abdominals peaks the internal pressure at the moment of the impact. This maneuver dramatically increases the muscular tension or force, for a fraction of a second," Pavel Tsatsouline explains. But the technique could leave you high if you try it the next time you test your bench max. Tsatsouline adds: "A bench lasts a lot longer than a punch. Try to ki-ya your way out of a big press, and the bar will collapse your sternum as surely as a karate chop." Why? Because once you've expelled all of the air, your intra-abdominal pressure will drop. So, instead, breathe out with a hiss or grunt that allows you to keep up your IAP throughout the rep. Who's got the loudest grunt? Tennis pro Maria Sharapova's loudest grunt was measured at 101 decibels.

Q: **What's a 360-degree brace?**

A: *First of all, here's what it's not. "It's definitely not a hollowing of your midsection, or trying to squeeze your belly button toward your spine," says Dr. Chad Waterbury, a high-performance physical therapist in Los Angeles. Waterbury goes on to say, "This is a correction I'm constantly making with inexperienced lifters. They need to expand their midsection to create 360 degrees of tension to support the spine and protect the discs from injury. Think of a water bottle that's full, and how it resists compression,*

> "Movement has two main attributes: stability and mobility. Your breathing impacts both, because each breath wields enormous influence over your ability to stabilize your core and spine—where all roads lead when it comes to strength training. All of the muscles involved in breathing play a role in postural stabilization. When those respiratory muscles fatigue your posture then compensate to create the movement needed for respiration that is not happening efficiently. And that's the reason why a person who breathes poorly limits the strength they can build up. Furthermore, since they can't develop it through a full range of motion, it also puts them at a greater risk for injury. So the way to have better stabilization, which allows for better lifts, is to work out your breathing and postural muscles."
>
> —Dr. Mark Cheng of K3 Combat Movement Systems[10]

---

10   Personal correspondence with Dr. Mark Cheng, October 18, 2018.

compared to an empty water bottle that's easy to crush."[12] So if you've ever heard the cue "navel to spine" in yoga class or "suck in that gut" from a bad gym teacher, or anyone else who's tried to teach you that sucking your gut inward is good for bearing load (lifting weights), go ahead and flush that from your memory.

Q: Just how big should a "Big Breath" be?

A: Let's imagine that you're going for a new PR on your back squat. How should you breathe? First, focus on the brace. You want the requisite tension in your body from head to toe. Second, exhale hard horizontally and inhale horizontally into your abdomen—not a Vertical Breath that lifts the chest. C. J. Murphy, a Boston-based strength coach, helps trainees achieve this by cueing them to "breathe through the back of your throat."[13] The iconic Louie Simmons (founder of Westside Barbell) advises lifters to pull in as much air as possible into a braced core prior to descending; whereas prominent Russian strength coach Boris Sheiko teaches lifters to inhale a much smaller mouthful of air. Often, you'll see lifters do both. Scientists at McGill's laboratory at the University of Waterloo studied how lung volume affects IAP, and they found that the optimal lies somewhere between the two approaches. Peak IAP came when lifters had inhaled to about 70 percent of their vital lung capacity or the total amount of air they could hold. So what does that mean to you? First, always brace. Second, always inhale before you start the lift. Third, how much air you take in to be your strongest will be a matter of trial and error. "I think it depends on the person," says Murphy. "We have found that some like to take more

The top three mistakes that Mike Ryan, E by Equinox MNR Programming Manager and Complex Tier X Manager, sees constantly:

1. Holding the breath (thoracic musculature rather than diaphragm).
2. Breathing in the "wrong" direction (e.g., inhaling when pushing a weight upward or exhaling fully prior to exertion).
3. Thinking "recovery time" is just a number of seconds that have to go by (often way more than needed as well). Breath inspires (no pun) the coexistence of mobility and stability allowing the body to rhythmically flow according to the joint by joint approach—if you can breathe in position, you don't own the position.

Their workouts get significantly better as soon as they breathe continuously, using the exhale while doing something effortful (regardless of if the direction is up or out), and then when recovering focusing on good inhales and exhales.

The coaching moment is getting them to understand the "why" behind purposeful breathing, whether to decrease tone or increase stability.[11]

---

11   Interview on April 22, 2019.

12   Personal correspondence, March 11, 2019.

13   Interview with Murphy, July 31, 2018.

air, and some are very good with the small puff. I think both are valid techniques. Sheiko lifters are insanely strong but Westside also produces insanely strong lifters."

Q: **Why do I get dizzy (or nosebleeds or feel like my head will pop) when I lift heavy?**

A: *Spectators at the 2012 Arnold Classic were treated to an incredible sight, but it got a little grisly. At that meet, powerlifting champion Brian Shaw deadlifted an astonishing 1,073 pounds. When Shaw ripped the bar and all eight giant truck tires stacked on it from the floor, blood burst out of his nose. It's for the same reason that other lifters will feel dizzy, burst blood vessels in their face, or even pass out while lifting heavy weights—an increase in blood pressure. Any time you close off the glottis, as you do in a Valsalva maneuver, blood pressure spikes. When you combine a closed glottis with flexed lower body muscles, the pressure forces blood upward into your head. Fighter pilots actually use this to their advantage: they flex their calves and thighs, and close their glottis to withstand the g-forces on fast sharp turns. If they didn't, the stronger force of gravity would push blood away from their brain and optic nerve, causing them to lose their vision and even pass out. "You're taught to say 'hick,' because when you say 'hick' it closes your glottis," explains Jay Consalvi, U.S. Navy fighter pilot and subject of the documentary* Speed and Angels.[14] *For pilots, the pressure is a lifesaver; for lifters, it can make for a gnarly end to an otherwise impressive lift.*

Q: **What's the difference between intrathoracic and intra-abdominal pressure?**

A: *Intrathoracic pressure refers to pressure in the thoracic cavity; i.e., the space above your diaphragm. Intra-abdominal pressure is pressure in the space below the diaphragm, the abdomen. Both of these forces support the spine. Intrathoracic pressure supports the upper back, while intra-abdominal pressure buttresses the lumbar spine and lower back.*

Q: **Where exactly does the air "go" when I inhale?**

---

14   Interview with Consalvi, August 26, 2018.

"Learning and practicing deep belly breathing does many things for our health and psyche, but when it comes to lifting, the most important thing it does is teach us to connect with our core. It teaches us to create tension and brace from the place we are meant to be stable. We cannot function, or lift, efficiently if we can't connect with our core."

—Michelle Martonick, competetive bodybuilder and powerlifter, and founder of Moxie in Motion in Los Angeles.

A: *It's a common misconception that air fills up the bottom of your lungs first, then moves upward to the top. In reality your lungs are a pressure system, with the air moving from high pressure to low. This means that on an inhale, the fresh air should move in all directions; however, often it does not if there is a restriction, such as a rigid torso or a taut diaphragm. If air encounters resistance while trying to go down into the alveoli-rich parts of your lungs, it will stay or flow upward into the apex of the lungs, which are less densely packed with air sacs.*

Q: **What about lifting, peeing, and prolapse?**

A: *CrossFit has never shied away from controversy, but the sport of fitness found itself in a true firestorm of criticism after releasing a 2013 video titled "Do You Pee During Workouts?" In the clip Rory McKernan asks multiple female competitors that exact question, and many answer "yes." The backlash from physiotherapists and other exercise professionals was swift and merciless. "This should not be celebrated," wrote Tracy Sher, MPT, CSCS. "Let's not make urinary leakage (and potential for increased pelvic organ prolapse) a goal to achieve as a marker of intensity!" she stressed on her Pelvic Guru site. What, then, makes a person pee—or prolapse—during a workout? It happens when the pressure inside their abdomen is greater than the muscles in their pelvic floor can hold. Basically, it's a messy way to discover that your pelvic floor is your weakest link or that it wasn't engaged at all. The solution: always remember that a good brace starts from the bottom. YouTube star Elliott Hulse brought much needed attention to the pelvic floor by coining the phrase "Breathe into your balls" on YouTube on March 22, 2013. The last thing you want to do is bear down on this important part of your body. Having a flexible and strong pelvic floor—the twenty muscles that are your "bicycle seat" and those that attach to it—are critically important to your lower back and pelvis health.*

Q: **Do smelling salts make you stronger?**

A: *Ever notice the little white packets on the sidelines in NFL games on TV? These capsules contain ammonia, which, when inhaled, irritates the membranes of the nose and lungs, thereby triggering an inhalation reflex. "This reflex alters the pattern of breathing, resulting in improved respiratory flow rates and possibly alertness," according to the National Institutes of Health. The result is an eye-opening jolt of alertness. Smelling salts are also popular with powerlifters for this reason. "The reason is because ammonia increases arousal, heart rate, all that sort of stuff," Dr. Mike T. Nelson,[15] an exercise physiologist and member of the American College of Sports Medicine, told STACK magazine. "When that happens, you are stronger from a gross motor standpoint. So if the task is to measure strength without much skill or technique, you do see an increase in that. The caveat is you see a decrease in fine motor ability, which is probably why you don't see Olympic lifters using smelling salts—their sport is more technique and skill-based. If you took a few whiffs of smelling salts and then tried to thread a needle, good frigging luck," he adds. So what does this mean for you? If your performance depends on brute strength alone, smelling salts might be helpful to you in a pinch. But if you're someone who in any way relies on fine motor control—like a baseball pitcher trying to slide the ball across just the lower corner of the plate, or a soccer player looking to sneak the ball past a goalie—smelling salts may actually be a hindrance. And if you do decide to use smelling salts, do so only occasionally: their eye-opening effect fades as you use them more, and irritating sensitive airways is not a good thing to do.*

Q: **What's the deal with people blowing up water bottles?**

A: *This is one of those Internet sensations that's been egged on by the Guinness Book of World Records, for some reason. The trend got its start in popular culture thanks to Oklahoma resident Brian Jackson, who says he got into hot water bottle bursting while recovering from a bad drug and alcohol problem. And while we applaud Jackson for turning his life around, the sport he's now popularized is seriously dangerous. "It can take up to 170 pounds of pressure to blow up [a hot water bottle]. It's like blowing up four car tires," Jackson said in a*

---

15   Hall, Brandon. "Are Smelling Salts Safe? An Eye-Opening Look at this Hype Up Method." STACK.com. November 20, 2015.

YouTube video. Yes, this requires a lot of strength; but also, "There's nothing to stop the air from coming back into my lungs," Jackson admits. And this could cause tremendous damage. If you want to show off how strong your breathing muscles are, use a balloon.

YOU ARE ASYMMETRICAL

Your heart takes up more space on the left side of your chest than the right. As a result, your left lung is smaller than your right lung.[16] Even your brain works asymmetrically, with the left side of your brain controlling the right side of your body (and vice versa). That's an extremely simplified version of the idea behind the work of Ron Hruska and the Postural Restoration Institute. Their institute is a big reason why you see so many high-profile athletes blowing into balloons during workouts, or placing their feet up on a wall after training. He says that many authorities fail to appreciate the powerful influence that the body's asymmetries have over us.

"You can open any textbook and are shown the right side is considered to be the same as the one on the left, but that's a complete misnomer," Hruska says.[17] He explains that as a result of our innate imbalances (which are natural and fine), we can develop a host of learned imbalances that aren't so great (such as "extended" posture, when a person has an anterior pelvic tilt). Anterior pelvic tilt and extended posture are common in athletic populations, and is sometimes called "hockey butt" for its prevalence

> I met with Juliana Malacarne at Don Saladino's gym Drive 495 in New York last summer. Juliana has won the Women's Physique Olympia four times in a row. I was so taken aback by her amazing ability to sense nuances within her body. "The left side moves more" she quipped, as I was teaching her about a Horizontal Breath. Rarely does someone have that very accurate sensation of the left side of their diaphragm being different than the right (the right side is thicker and less mobile because of the liver).

16   Tsai, Jang-Zern et al. "Left-Right Asymmetry in Spectral Characteristics of Lung Sounds Detected Using a Dual-Channel Auscultation System in Healthy Young Adults"; and Anderson, Robert H. et al. "Cardiac anatomy revisited." https://www.ncbi.nlm.nih.gov/pubmed/28590447.

17   Interview with Ron Hruska and Jen Platt, Postural Restoration Institute, December 19, 2018.

among players of that sport. PRI's 90/90 Hip Lift with Balloon is an exercise that can help athletes restore a more neutral position, improving breathing and decreasing the likelihood of back pain.

12

MASTERING TENSION FOR MAXIMUM MUSCLE

TEN POUNDS OF MUSCLE

No strength coach would ever draw up a plan that trained every part of the body except the left glute. Nor would they ever sign off on a program that trained every part of the body except the right shoulder. Yet this is exactly what happens when athletes do not train their breathing muscles, and there are a lot more of those muscles than most people realize. A 180-pound athlete, for example, has 52 pounds of actual muscle (bones, fat, and bodily organs make up the rest).

While this is the beginning of a conversation about the formal integration of the role of the diaphragm and respiratory muscles in training, the topics on which top trainers agree include:

1. Developing your diaphragmatic awareness. Physical therapist and sports performance specialist Dr. John Rusin has his clients develop better kinesthetic awareness of their diaphragms by lying on the floor facedown and pushing the floor away with each inhale. It's called Crocodile Breathing.[1]

2. Addressing your lifting posture. Once you understand how Vertical Breathing has been a factor in your bad posture, you can use Horizontal Breathing to fix it. Trainers may correct this at the beginning of a workout through a core workout that involves planks, Dead Bugs, or 90/90 Breathing on the floor (which means your hips and knees are both bent at

---

1   For more on this technique, see: Rusin, John. "Fix Your Breathing, Build More Muscle," t-nation.com, June 7, 2017.

90 degrees), and other moves meant to restore a neutral spine. "Just by getting guys back to neutral, pretty good things happen," points out Eric Cressey. Those "good things" include better stability at the core.[2]

3. Building a better brace. Your brace is what protects you from injury when you lift. In this chapter we'll talk at length about breathing and bracing. The most commonly used brace is called the Valsalva maneuver. Technically speaking, a Valsalva occurs when you exhale against a closed glottis. "In Russia, we say the Valsalva is an exhalation that has not happened," Pavel Tsatsouline points out.[3] The Valsalva maneuver increases intra-abdominal pressure, which in turn "stiffens" and stabilizes the spine, creating more explosive strength.

4. Breathing *while* you brace. While the Valsalva is great for 1-rep maxes and other all-out efforts, not every set is so extreme or so short. Contrast this to when you "breathe behind the shield": your torso muscles are engaged enough to protect you but not so much that it's impossible to inhale and exhale. In fact, skilled practitioners can even talk while they maintain "the shield." To demonstrate how this works, TRX Rip Trainer inventor Pete Holman has been known to speak to workshops while also being punched in the stomach by an attendee.[4]

> "Breathing is the first movement. You need to organize around the spine for the best shape that is available to it, considering the pelvic floor and diaphragm. We are a system that is built around the spine, and you have to respect the central nervous system. Our body will work around it (through compensation) because it's an extraordinary problem-solving machine. The brain is the most sophisticated structure in the known universe. Focus on breath integrity—peak mechanical ventilation and the radial abdominal contractile field—so you can create real stability instead of reflexive stability."
>
> — Kelly Starrett, *On Becoming a Supple Leopard*

---

2   On YouTube, October 24, 2003.

3   Interview with Tsatsouline, August 17, 2018.

4   To actually see this, check out his podcast "Breathing Behind the Shield." Holman points out that "You can also harness your breath to match the exertion you are generating; for example, a fast, hard strike like a punch gets a fast, hard breath, while a slower, and more grinding effort like an overhead press is best paired with a slower exhalation that allows you to retain more intra-abdominal pressure."

TO BREATHE OR NOT TO BREATHE: THE SPINAL STIFFNESS SPECTRUM

A part from the obvious, *stiffness* is not a word that conjures a positive image. You think of someone who is not graceful on the dance floor, an uncomfortable outfit, being overly hair-sprayed, or having joint pain. Spinal stiffness, on the other hand, is specific to weight lifting literature, and is something you very much want, especially when you know how to adjust the amount of stiffness to the need.

The first question that springs to mind is: Should you breathe at all when you lift? A held breath increases internal pressure while allowing you to generate more force, while breathing makes for more fluid movement and is, consequently, a source of instability.

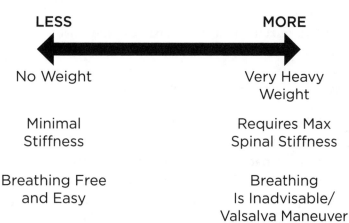

SPINAL STIFFNESS NEEDED

LESS   **MORE**

No Weight   Very Heavy Weight

Minimal Stiffness   Requires Max Spinal Stiffness

Breathing Free and Easy   Breathing Is Inadvisable/ Valsalva Maneuver

Figure 12.1

Imagine a spectrum of activities that range from no load (weight) on the far left, to those involving extremely heavy loads on the far right. For those far right activities, like powerlifting, your goal should be to achieve maximum stiffness in the spine. A person who has several hundred pounds sitting atop their back wants as much tension in their midsection as possible; otherwise their spine would buckle (and catastrophe would be the result).

At the very far left would be exercises that involve no load whatsoever and lots of movement. An example is distance running, in which you can take several steps per breath and don't need to maintain tension throughout your core the whole time. In fact, doing so would be a waste of energy.

In your spectrum each activity in between has a different degree of the proximal (core) stiffness required for optimum movement. Other than muscular strength, the most direct control you have over your core stiffness is through your breathing. Dr. Stuart McGill says that a good rule of thumb is: "The greater the load, the more you shouldn't breathe during activity. Powerlifters do not breathe under exertion and interestingly great sprinters just take mini-sips of air."

The majority of the movements you make in sports and in the gym fall somewhere between the two extremes. Being aware of them and making informed choices is what keeps you strong and injury-free.

We've talked about biomechanical and anatomical breathing before, but let's delve a little deeper on the topic.

BIOMECHANICAL BREATHING

For the purposes of strength training, most people should be using biomechanical breathing. What does that mean in simple terms? Well, the easiest way to remember relies on a simple tip from Boston-based coach and owner of CORE collective, Tony Gentilcore: "Exhale when you exert effort. This is true whether you are pushing the weight away from or pulling it toward you."[5] For the specifics of what you do

The respiratory muscles don't just move air in and out of the body; they also create stability and, broadly speaking, stability creates strength. "In the eyes of our clinicians and trainers, nothing is more crucial than the maintenance of trunk stability," says Dr. Kathy Dooley, rehabilitative chiropractor and cofounder of Catalyst S.P.O.R.T. in New York. "Trunk stability is the platform for all human movement."

5   Email correspondence with Gentilcore, August 1, 2018.

when, go back to our stiffness spectrum: during a very heavy lift, you may let out a grunt only at the sticking point. Use breathing not to extend or contract your body but rather to encourage good mechanics. Biomechanical Breathing means you use the breath hold for stiffness and explosiveness. The explosiveness or more dramatic effort happens on the exhale.

This contrasts with Anatomical Breathing, which focuses on your spine movement. As we explained in chapter seven, if you are extending, you are inhaling; if you are flexing, you are exhaling. This breathing is used when you lift little or no weight, and are focusing on the integrity of the movement. Anatomical Breathing is also called Reverse Breathing because it is the opposite of biomechanical.

SPECIFIC PRO ADVICE FOR SPECIFIC MOVEMENTS

Now, moving forward, let's get the specifics for each of the main types of exercises from the pros.

BENCH PRESS

"Do you really 'own' the posture," asks Rob Wilson, Art of Breath cofounder, "or are you just muscling your way through it." In an interview this year he told me the answer: "Only if you can breathe well in it." One of his favorites that hits home is hanging from a chinning bar and blowing up a balloon.

"Hold your breath to stay tight and keep as much tension as possible for the entirety of the repetition," instructs Jim Smith, CPPS and owner of Diesel Strength.[6] If you are struggling to get past the sticking point, you can let out a hiss on the upward press. Release and reset the breath after each rep, but only after you've achieved lockout.

MILITARY OR OVERHEAD PRESS

Here you'd use what Dan John calls the *psst!* breath, which sounds exactly as it looks: as if you were trying to get someone's attention in a library. In a *psst!* breath, you take

---

6   Email correspondence with Smith, August 5, 2018.

a big inhale, brace your midsection, and start the lift. With each exertion, you take only a tiny bit of air in and out, making the *psst!* noise. You can either hold your breath or inhale slightly through your nose during the lowering phase. "You're basically keeping all that air in your body to keep the pressure in, but you have to breathe," John says.[7]

PULL-UPS OR CHIN-UPS

Hang from the bar, feet slightly in front of your body—your shoulder blades will be "packed" or drawn down and in. "Start with taking a breath of air to 'set' everything, and then exhale when you pull," Gentilcore says. "At the top you'll want to get a sip of air before you descend (to ensure you maintain core/full-body tension), and then repeat the whole process for subsequent reps." He recommends breathing and resetting on each rep, but adds, "I can see where, if someone is performing higher rep sets, they may hold their breath for a rep or two before resetting."[8]

SQUAT

Here's a step-by-step guide: 1) Inhale and tense your middle to "set" your brace. 2) Hold that breath as you lower to the bottom of the rep, then continue to hold it on the way back up at least until you reach the sticking point. 3) Either let out a grunt or just continue to hold until you reach the top of the rep. Exhaling out a spoonful and rebracing will release a bit of pressure, and that can be a good thing: "There are a few times when I've blacked out under the bar where I think I wouldn't have if I'd let some of that air out," says C. J. Murphy, a strongman competitor, powerlifting champion, and creator of Total Performance Method. And on sub-maximal efforts where you are performing two or more reps, you can either breathe and reset at the top or hold your breath, although Murphy recommends not holding your breath for much more than a triple.

---

7   Interview with John, July 27, 2018.

8   Email correspondence with Gentilcore, August 1, 2018.

DEADLIFT

You have two opportunities to breathe before you deadlift. One is while you are standing over the bar; the other is after you've dropped down to take your grip. According to Jesse Burdick of PowerWod.com, breathing at the top is an option that only advanced lifters should pursue. Nearly everyone else should take their last big lower-body breath after gripping the bar, but before they start the pull. "Grab the bar first, then breathe with your hips high and while you have more space," he says in a blog post on Diesel Strength & Conditioning's website. "Then drop into place, setting the spring and creating tension. Then you pull the weight."

> "The Open-scissor Effect: Failing to breathe and brace properly causes the ribs to flare and the back to overarch. This may be the most common squatting mistake—people think that because their back is arched (rather than rounded) that their low back is safe. But it's actually in too much extension rather than neutral. Learning to pull the ribs down, tuck the pelvis under slightly, so that the torso and hips are aligned and neutral, is critical."[9]
>
> — Sean Hyson, author of *The Men's Health Encyclopedia of Muscle: Everything You Need to Know to Build the Body You Want*

KETTLEBELL SWINGS

In his book, *Kettlebell Simple & Sinister*, Tsatsouline relates that his StrongFirst group uses biomechanical breathing (i.e., exhaling on the upswing) because their goal is to develop strength, and exhaling with the exertion allows them to generate more force than inhaling. "Like in a punch, you get extra power with the help of the reflex when you exhale sharply and forcefully with your abdomen. In addition, you squeeze the carbon dioxide from the bottoms of the lungs. This is critical for going the distance because when you start sucking wind, it is generally not from the lack of oxygen but from a buildup of CO_2."[10]

PLANKS

Planking is a slightly different animal; you have to learn to take small breaths while maintaining a brace in your midsection. "In a high threshold strategy, where everything is locked down, you're

---

9   Interview, December 18, 2018.

10 Interview, Tsatsouline, August 17, 2018.

probably going to use the Valsalva Maneuver," says trainer Mike Robertson.[11] If you are struggling to breathe while planking, put your elbows up on a bench. This lightens the load, so that you can breathe more normally.

SIT-UPS

TACFIT creator and coach Scott Sonnon has been integrating the breath in workouts for decades. His "Be Breathed" method on sit-ups goes as follows: inhale as you lower your torso toward the floor, then use the exhale to help propel your body up and forward. Release all of the air you can at the top, then inhale and start the descent for your next rep.

LEG PRESSES

The advantage you have when leg pressing is that you don't have to maintain max tension throughout your core owing to the fact that there isn't a weight on your back that would put it at risk. So you can breathe a bit more freely. Here Dan John recommends using what he calls the *"Choo-Choo"* breath—although it's less like the noise of a train in the distance and more like the whooshing sound you'd hear at the ocean. You take big inhalations as you lower the weight, and powerful exhalations when you press. "You're turning your body into a piston," John explains.[12]

---

11   Email correspondence with Robertson, August 8, 2018.
12   Interview with John, July 27, 2018.

LOADED CARRIES

A loaded carry is what you require to get something heavy from point A to point B. Loaded carries give you the ability to generate and then control tension. Carries require you to generate a brace, and then move with it. "What I like about loaded carries is they force you to breathe correctly. You don't have a choice," John points out. Broadly speaking, there are three types (listed in order of ascending difficulty).

FARMER'S CARRIES

When you carry an equal amount of weight in each hand, but you don't want to limply support each weight so that they balance between your palm and fingers. "The Farmer's Carry is a moving plank," John stresses.

ASYMMETRICAL CARRIES

When you carry different loads in each hand, or carry a weight in one hand while leaving the other empty, which is a move called the Suitcase Carry.

BEAR HUG CARRIES

"What fails first, your muscles or your breathing? Your breathing," Julien Pineau of StrongFit explains. Pineau uses sandbags as an example of how Cyclical Breathing—a breath that supports your rhythm—is key (and also clears out lactate faster). How? Take two steps while inhaling, and then exhaling on the next two steps.[13]

When you hold a weight against your body with both arms.

"A Farmer's Walk teaches you to have proper posture," John added in an interview we had with him: "You'll notice that you probably almost flow through an 'ohm' kind of breathing. You can get away with breathing out through your chest, but you're better off breathing lower, especially as the distance of the carry gets farther and farther."

Surprising as it may seem, doing a Suitcase

---

13   You can hear more about Pineau and pain caves, pythons, and shark fins on Mike Bledslow, Doug Larson, and Chris Moore's podcast *Barbell Shrugged* (episode 190).

Carry with an 80-pound dumbbell will actually be harder for most people than carrying two 75-pound dumbbells in a Farmer's Carry. Even though the Farmer's Carry requires you to move more weight overall, your body has to generate greater tension in order to be able to carry the single dumbbell in one hand. (Note that this requires you to brace your midsection so that your hips and shoulders are relatively level. You don't want to have the weight pull you over to one side.) "Because you have to brace the opposite side in the Suitcase Carry, that's going to teach you anaconda strength quickly," John notes.

That internal pressure is even more important when you have to hold the weight against your body in order to move with it. "If you're doing a Bear Hug Carry with something as light as 80 pounds, you know, after about 20 steps, if you don't have internal pressure, you just start to break down," John adds.

Learning to generate this tension—and breathe through it—will carry over to every exercise you do in the gym. That's why John teaches Farmer's Walks on day one for any new trainee. "If you can't master tension, then we can't put load on you."

EXERCISE

HARDSTYLE BREATHING

Here's a breathing/bracing drill that famed strength coach Pavel Tsatsouline has termed Hardstyle Breathing,

---

14   Made popular by Steve Maxwell. https://www.maxwellsc.com.

DAN JOHN'S RECOVERY BREATHING LADDER

The concept of breathing ladders is credited to physical therapist Steve McNamara.[14] In a breathing ladder, you match the number of breaths you can take during your rest period with the number of reps performed during a set. The number of breaths you take while moving is deliberate; the number of breaths you take between reps is deliberate (professional CrossFit athlete Rich Froning is known for timing his rest intervals with his breath count). So if you were to perform 10 squats or presses, you'd take 10 controlled breaths for recovery. Your rest ends when you complete the tenth breath. Repeat for a set time interval. John explains: "OK, here's your workout, for the next five minutes, you're going to do 10 goblet squats, then you start up when you finish 10 breaths." And then he clarifies: "For me, the winner is the person who does the least number of squats. This pattern naturally encourages you to lengthen your breaths, because longer breaths mean longer recovery. You're getting punished—literally punished—for breathing fast. It helps you master breath control right away." The result is that you learn how to control your breathing in stressful situations, a technique that carries over into many other aspects of life. In addition, it is used in recovery breathing. "What's going to happen there is that, after stress, I know how to cool down. I'm just going to count my breaths," John concludes.

and after the first few rounds you'll know how it earned the name.

1. Place your hands on your abs and obliques.
2. Breathe diaphragmatically into the lower body.
3. Engage your pelvic floor. Tsatsouline cues this by asking people to imagine they are trying to "prevent both kinds of nature's call."
4. Place your tongue against your teeth.
5. Squeeze your abs while exhaling in short bursts. Make a hiss noise with each exhalation. Readjust and retense your body after each exhale, hard.
6. Exhale for five pulses or until you blow out all the air. Do not tense your face, neck, or traps; keep all the tension below your armpits.
7. Relax. Do not do another set for at least several minutes to avoid getting light-headed.

BREATHING FOR OLYMPIC LIFTING

In Olympic lifting the bar spends most of its time in one of three places: on the floor, above your head, or on your throat. None of them are ideal for breathing, which is why California Strength coach Glenn Pendlay recommends that most people breathe before starting a rep, and then not worry about it. "Normally, you're not breathing in or out when you pull," Pendlay says, adding: "You're certainly not going to breathe in. There are some people who let a little bit of breath out as they pull. That's fairly rare, though. Most of the time, during the pull you're going to hold your breath."[15]

With the bar at your throat, your goal is to fully "catch" your breath by whatever means necessary. Then you press the bar over-head with a short, forceful exhale. Once the bar is overhead, you have another chance to catch your breath. "For me, it's just finding that good stacked position where your bones and joints are holding the weight, not your muscles," says four-time CrossFit Games champ

---

15　Check out his website, CaliforniaStrength.com for more details.

Mat Fraser in *Men's Health*.[16] "It's obviously not weightless, but you aren't straining to hold it up."

BUILDING THE SHIELD

Here's a technique from Dr. McGill's book, *Ultimate Back Fitness and Performance*, that ensures you train the diaphragm directly. Perform an exercise that makes you breathe heavily: run, ride an Airdyne, smash some battle ropes, you name it. Go hard for a minute or so. Once you are breathing rapidly, drop down and hold a side plank. Why a side plank? Because in order to maintain that position, all of those muscles throughout the trunk that might ordinarily assist with respiration have to fire in order to stabilize the spine. If they didn't, you'd fall out of the bridge. That forces all of the work of breathing onto the diaphragm. "You build 'the shield' through core stiffness, and behind that shield the diaphragm becomes a pump," explains McGill.

Whatever sort of lifting you are doing, if you are using a dysfunctional Vertical Breath, you aren't breathing in a strong, biomechanically sound way—either on inhale or exhale. Consequently, you are going to experience fatigue faster and, more important, put yourself at risk for injury. The concept of stacking your body correctly doesn't make sense with a Vertical Breath. Your breathing is not fueling your muscles as efficiently as it could. Research clearly documents that your balance and stability become of secondary importance when respiratory muscles experience fatigue. Your intermittent

> Pavel Tsatsouline, the former Soviet Special Forces physical training instructor, uses a technique he learned in diving school called Straw Breathing in order to teach people proper lower-body breathing. "Lie down on the ground, put a drinking straw in your mouth, pinch off your nose, and just breathe. When you can comfortably do that, line up two straws and make it longer. Then go to three straws, which is usually enough." This method increases the amount of "dead space" you have to breathe through in order to get air. The straw becomes an extension of that. "The straw forces you to inhale very deep into your abdomen—and to exhale very completely from the bottom of your lungs."[17]

---

16   Mestel, Spenser. "Crush This Grueling CrossFit Workout With Help From the Fittest Man on Earth." *Men's Health*, March 26, 2018.

17   Interview with Tsatsouline, August 17, 2018. This technique is also described in Tsatsouline's book, *Kettlebell Simple & Sinister*.

necessary breath hold and, subsequently, less-than-optimal Vertical Breath (because it takes up more energy than it produces) are inefficient. That one dramatic "up" breath you take from time to time is more of a ritual than a refuel. That breath doesn't decompress and reset your spine, and your bracing lasts way too long into your day.

DO THIS NOW

1 squat	1 breath (one full inhale and exhale)
2 squats	2 breaths
3 squats	3 breaths
4 squats	4 breaths
5 squats	5 breaths

Go up in reps, then come down. Meaning get to 5 (or 10 or 20 depending on weight and your strength), then go back down the "ladder" finishing at 1:1.

Don't train for time. Focus is on the breath and the integrity of movement.

You can also do 1 rep: 10 breaths to recover, or any variation of that type.

13

APPLIED STRENGTH: HOW TO BREATHE DURING THE MAJOR LIFTS

THE GYM HIGH FIVE

Here is the summary of the breathing information you've now mastered.

1. Your inhale is efficient. It gives you intrathoracic pressure, protects your spine, and makes for explosiveness. In addition, you use it to recover quickly and completely between lifts or sets.
2. You've reframed your breathing: your entire middle (abdominothoracic) "softens" and expands, while the exhale narrows, along with your ribs. It makes sense, for it's where the largest, densest part of your lungs is found.
3. Your obliques and pelvic floor are your new BFFs. Find them. Hang out with them. If you are ripped and jacked, your abs are not, meaning that on the inhale they should soften. Otherwise, they are just strangling you and thereby encouraging stiff neck and shoulder muscles (because you are using these as primary breathing muscles).
4. You do not brace continually. Before, between bracing and peacocking, you were barely breathing, which meant you were low on fuel and your lower back was unhappy. You know better now.
5. You decompress your spine between lifts, and refuel by inhaling and widening your middle. When you do that, your diaphragm sends blood and gives your discs space. Feel how the "rebrace" feels stronger afterward. Notice how a Horizontal Breath cues a tighter brace.

TARGETED BREATHING
FOR STRENGTH TRAINING

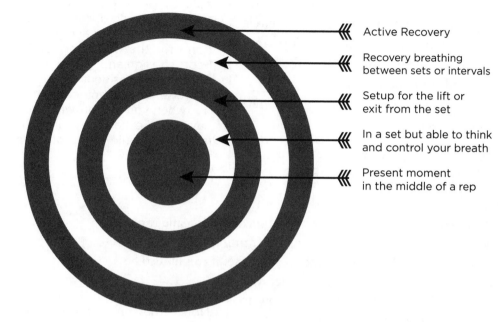

Active Recovery

Recovery breathing
between sets or intervals

Setup for the lift or
exit from the set

In a set but able to think
and control your breath

Present moment
in the middle of a rep

TARGETED BREATHING

Let's return to the analogy of an archery target we used in an earlier chapter. Several circles surround a deep red bull's-eye in the middle. Each circle represents a different moment in your strength training session. How conscious you are of your breathing will be different at each circle.

- The bull's-eye represents the moment when you are in the middle of a rep. You are absolutely in the present moment.
- The first circle out from the bull's-eye is the moment when you are in a set but able to think and control your breath. This encompasses points such as the moment just before you start a rep when you perform your Valsalva, or when you are trying to grunt through a sticking point.
- The second circle represents your setup for the lift or exit from the set. Here's where you do things such as take your deep inhale and set an initial brace to get under the bar, or

hold that brace/other tension until you fully rack the weight.

- The next circle is your recovery breathing between sets or intervals. This circle is very important to your performance when you are getting closer to the bull's-eye and your goal.
- The farthest circle out is your active recovery.

BRACE + HORIZONTAL BREATH = BETTER BRACE AND MORE AIR

"On the power production strength side, you have to be able to really do a sweet-ass Valsalva. Small doses of high stressor, 1 to 3 reps and you are done for the day." Bert Sorin, Scottish Highland games competitor and president of Sorinex Exercise Equipment continues, ". . . when you are throwing, you have rapid exhaling—your focus is on contractile speed of large muscles groups."

Once you are able to continuously perform a B-IQ "A" on demand (meaning a perfect location of motion and range of motion), then you can start practicing breathing from a different part of your body while keeping other parts tense. It might also be that the situation or exercise doesn't let you breathe normally. Do you really know how to breathe "through your back"? Or from your sides? Call yourself out when you revert to an inefficient Vertical Breath or just hold. The Hammer Strength Seated Row is an example of breathing through your back and narrowing on the exhale.[1] You don't have to worry about balance, your stomach and chest are pressed against the front pad, and on the inhale your arms stretch forward. While the aim is to exhale on effort and engage your lats and back, use the inhale rather than just considering it the moment

Notice the stark difference between inhaling vertically and bracing, and inhaling horizontally and bracing. When you unbrace in order to breathe horizontally, your brace feels stronger. In fact, it is. You have recruited your core muscles by unbracing first. The breath you are taking is also significantly bigger (up to 4 to 6 times what an upper-body breath can be).

---

1   If you walk into Gold's Gym Venice and see a man whose lats span two postal codes, it's probably Super Heavyweight Power Bodybuilder Doug Fruchey. Doug was the one who brought the beauty of the Hammer Strength Seated Row machine and the breath to my attention. Despite his huge mass, Doug has excellent Abdominothoracic Respiratory Flexibility and a perfect Horizontal Breath; he has an "A" grade on his B-IQ.

in between your rep. And if you love the intricacies of this, the back breath lets you stretch further (more efficient movement) and keeps you better oxygenated (for more and heavier reps).

> *"Breath facilitates movement. Movement facilitates breath. Breath facilitates stability. Stability facilitates movement. It's just one big circle."*

—*Sue Falsone*, Bridging the Gap from Rehab to Performance

THE GOLD STANDARD: LOCOMOTIVE PAIRING AND STAYING HONEST

Full integration of efficient breathing rests on two pillars:

1. Keeping your breathing LOM and ROM as precise as you can. Stay honest. Unfortunately, most people will unconsciously switch to a Vertical Breath when faced with resistance, be it nasal or from a resistance device. When you are training, keep the focus so that your breathing form will stay true. Once in competition, go all out and focus on the gold.
2. Making sure your "locomotive pairing" is correct; form and stability are key.
   a. Decide if your movement is mechanical or anatomical, or a combination thereof.
   b. Hold your breath for only short amounts of time. Breathe actively in between.
   c. Know how to brace efficiently (circumferentially and including the pelvic floor).
   d. Grunt on exhale because it helps rebrace with explosiveness.
   e. Actively recover, reset, and oxygenate between sets in order to fight fatigue.

FREQUENTLY ASKED QUESTIONS

Q: How long before a Vertical Breath stops feeling better than a Horizontal one?

A: *A Vertical Breath might feel natural to you because it's such an in-grained habit, but you will not be getting enough air and it can con-tribute to your fatigue and risk of injury. Now that you know that intellectually, it will trump your going back to a Vertical Breath. Sure, you might raise your shoulders when you sigh from time to time out of habit, but notice that you now catch yourself. Notice how a truly an-atomically congruous, efficient breath heightens the awareness you have of the middle of your body—one that you never had before.*

Q: **What do you mean by "a Horizontal Breath cues a tighter brace"?**

A: *When you are a Vertical Breather, your inhale is up and your exhale is down. Down leads you to brace in a downward motion, which is not as efficient, and also strains your pelvic floor. Now inhale horizontally, then brace horizontally, squeezing your pelvic floor, then your middle. You are more apt to conjure a 360-degree brace. In ad-dition, now your pelvic floor contraction makes for a better brace since you are not just "leaning" on the muscles and feeling them bulge (and even-tually herniate).*

For jumping and throwing exercises, athletes should inhale before the action and exhale while performing it. Tudor Bompa stipulates: "During isometric contractions athletes should hold their breathing only a very short time or not at all. Have the muscles contract; the natural tendency is to hold one's breath, but athletes should concentrate breathing throughout the contraction." Regarded as the father of sports periodization theory, Bompa stressed training with variable loads throughout the year in order to achieve optimal performance. For more on jumping, read Derek Hansen and Steve Kennedy's *Plyometric Anatomy*.

Q: **I use a belt. How does this change the breathing for me?**

A: *Have you noticed how powerlifters who always use a belt tend to have thicker waists? They actu-ally have good horizontal inhales. But here's where things get ugly: their exhales are terrible—usually still "down" on a Vertical Breath—and they are full of residual air. Here's the Rx: if you lift with a belt, work diligently on your exhale. You may not ever "hollow out" when lifting, but make sure you can do it to exhale the rest of the time.*

Q: **What is the breathing fascia connection?**

A: *Owing to the fact that Vertical Breathing draws in less air with each breath, you need to breathe faster. And since each breath has been* relegated to your upper chest, you overuse your shoulder and other accessory muscles, consequently developing imbalances and trigger points throughout your fascia. According to Josh Stolz, fitness trainer, motor learning and movement expert and founder of TheStolzMovement, "The fascia is like a sheet out of a dryer; it gets super crinkly and needs to be smoothed out. The tension of sitting, fatigue, and terrible posture 'wrinkles' it, so to speak. Breathing and meditation 'iron' out the wrinkles and send a positive relaxing lengthening signal."[2]

"The spine slightly extends when we inhale and flexes when we exhale, which allows healthy dynamic disc movement. Intervertebral discs have no direct blood supply and rely on this movement for nutrition and oxygen via a process called diffusion. Simply put, efficient diaphragmatic breathing means your intervertebral discs are getting access to more blood flow," explains Brad M. Gilden, PT, DPT, CFMT, FAAOMPT, FFMT, CSCS. "You want more spinal disk movement paired with breathing in both directions which is critical in keeping discs healthy."[3]

Q: I keep getting told to "exhale and let go, relax" but this is wrong, right?

A: When you exhale, your heart rate slows slightly. If you inhale horizontally, then the exhale is a recoil (which does not happen with a Vertical Breath!). The cue to "let it go" refers to your unwanted thoughts along with the exhale of the breath, but it's been misunderstood as a cue to relax your body. The problem with telling a Vertical Breather this is that you are reinforcing paradoxical breathing, which is an extreme Vertical Breath. The bottom line is that your exhale will be completely inefficient, meaning, there will too much residual air in your body. (A sponge should narrow when squeezing the water out, right?)

Q: Exhaling and narrowing feels like the opposite of what I want to do, why?

A: Usually when you "pose," you'll inhale, puff up your chest and lats, and narrow your belly. I am asking you to do the opposite, which is anatomically more efficient. While inhale and "pose" look great on stage, it's the opposite of how you should be breathing in real life.

---

2   Interview, May 2019.

3   Interview with Gilden, February 2019.

EXERCISES

The classic instructions to inhale through your nose, and exhale through your mouth apply here, unless you are taking mouthfuls of air to rebrace or are doing sets and need to move to a mouth-mouth "gear."[4]

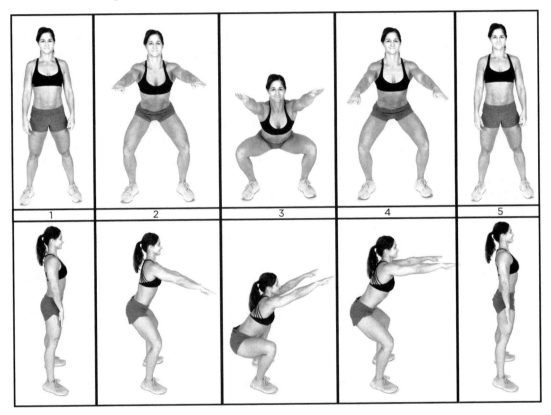

AIR SQUAT MECHANICAL INSTRUCTIONS

1. Establish your stance with your feet slightly turned out, "screwing" your feet into the ground.
2. Reach your hamstrings back, keeping your shins as vertical as possible. Press your knees out laterally and start lowering into the bottom position.
3. Rise out of the bottom position in reverse.

---

4   See Kelly Starrett's *On Becoming a Supple Leopard* for more details.

4. As you stand up, your shoulder girdle and upper back are muscularly activated.
5. Reclaim a stable top position by squeezing your glutes.

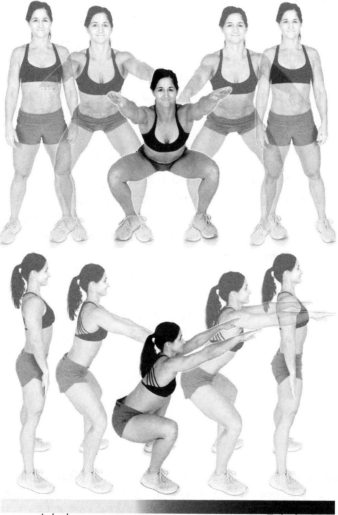

Inhale   Exhale

BREATHING INSTRUCTIONS

1. Before starting a set, make sure you relax your body and take big horizontal decompressing breaths as you get into your stance.
2. Inhale as you move downward.
3. This is not a huge breath, but rather an evenly paced 360-degree inhale that will help with the momentum of the exhale.
4. Transition to exhale.
5. Exhale audibly as you ascend.
6. The end of the exhale should correspond with the glute contraction that occurs at the top of this movement.

NOTE

Another approach you could take with air squats (as well as other bodyweight moves like push-ups and sit-ups) is to alternate how you breathe on different sets. For example, if you were going to perform 10 sets of 10 air squats, exhale on the way up for 5 of those sets, and then inhale on the way up for 5 sets.[5]

---

5   If you are doing them to "grease the groove" for sets of squats with heavier resistance, you'll want to exhale on the way up. That's because an exhale on the way up mimics what you'll do when you are under load. But if you are performing bodyweight squats as a conditioning exercise or doing a high number of them for time, you may be better off inhaling on the way up. Why? "That extra pressure from the diaphragm is gonna help you come up faster," says Pavel Tsatsouline. "This works great for endurance situations," such as the 300 air squats you perform in a Murph in CrossFit.

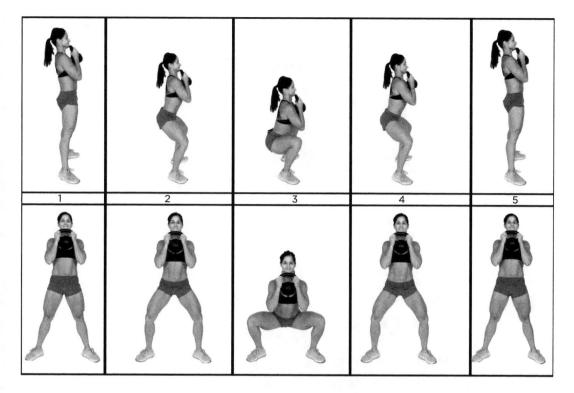

GOBLET SQUAT MECHANICAL INSTRUCTIONS

1. Position your feet just outside your shoulder width.
2. Bend your knees while trying to keep your shins as vertical as possible and driving your knees out.
3. Stop when your thighs are parallel to the floor.
4. Push to ascend.
5. Come back to the starting position.

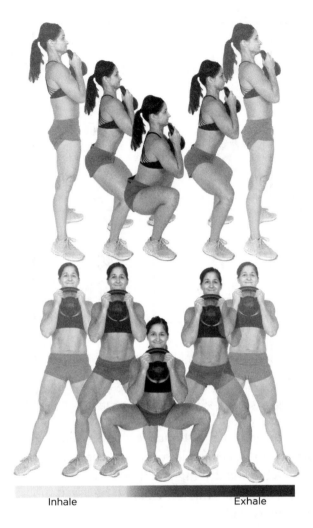

Inhale   Exhale

BREATHING INSTRUCTIONS

1. Start inhale.
2. Finish inhale.
3. Hold.
4. Start to exhale. (You may let out an audible mouthful of air to help ascend.)
5. Finish exhale as you return to standing. (If the weight is heavy and you are doing reps, you may find you don't fully exhale until your set is done and you have released the weight.)

NOTE

The tension needed to hold the kettlebell in front of your body will help keep your breath low. Start to notice how your breathing is more circumferential (lateral and back) because of this. You should feel your sides move on the inhale.

TROUBLESHOOT

You might find you are holding your breath two seconds from the middle of the descent to the middle of the ascent because of the weight and balance that this requires.

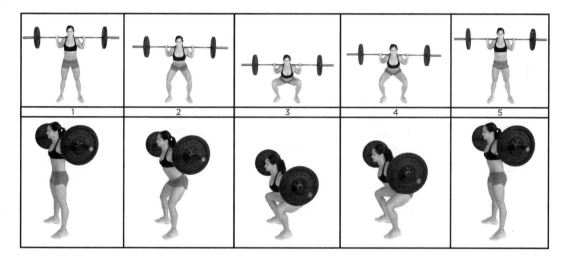

BACK SQUAT MECHANICAL INSTRUCTIONS

1. Place the bar evenly on your back in either the high bar (on your upper traps) or low bar (along the posterior deltoids/ mid traps) position. Tighten your upper back. Stand up to lift the barbell off the rack and carefully take a few small steps backward to get into position for the exercise. Once you get into position, set your feet in your preferred stance.

2. Press hips back slightly then down as the knees bend to lower into the squat, while keeping your core tight and your back flat. As you lower, imagine that you're spreading the ground apart with your feet and pulling your butt to your heels.

3. Your knees should track outward directly over your toes.
    Continue until your thighs are parallel to the ground.
4. Drive through your midfoot and extend your hips and knees
    explosively.
5. Stand up completely in the same position in which you started.

BREATHING INSTRUCTIONS

1. Inhale and brace once the bar is wedged on your back, and
    feels solid.
2. While holding breath and bracing, descend.
3. Keep the brace and breathhold at the bottom.
4. At the "sticking point," you may grunt or exhale slightly and
    rebrace to help power the completion of the move.
5. Exhale for momentum to finish the movement.
6. Inhale a medium-size breath, brace, go again.

NOTE

If the weight is not heavy, you may do two reps for each breath.
An alternative is lung packing a gulp or two after picking the bar
up. Do not fully exhale at the sticking point (or while you have the
bar on your back).

TROUBLESHOOT

Between sets, take good deep Horizontal Breaths. This is important for energy and unbracing your body so you can rebrace
tightly. Remember fatigue brought about by bad breathing can
lead to injury.

BENCH PRESS MECHANICAL INSTRUCTIONS

1. Lie underneath the bar; it should be at your collarbone.
2. Before lifting the weight out of the rack, pull your shoulder
    blades together, activate lats and upper back, setting your
    shoulders in a stable position.
3. Lift the weight out of the rack and align the bar over your
    shoulders.

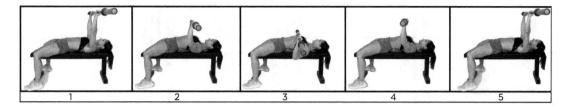

4. Keeping your shoulder blades pulled back, lower the weight to your chest.
5. Extend your elbows and reestablish the start position.

BREATHING INSTRUCTIONS

1. Take a big breath before you lie down.
2. Inhale while your shoulder blades and hips are in position. Exhale.
3. Inhale and hold briefly while lifting the weight out of the rack and aligning. Exhale.
4. Inhale as you lower.
5. Exhale as you push the bar up.

NOTE

Any time the weight is out of the rack, you do not fully inhale or exhale. Your big breaths come only after the weight is fully racked.

TROUBLESHOOT

At step 2 you can think of the inhale as one where your body expands "forward"—it helps set your shoulder blades and hips in a stable position.

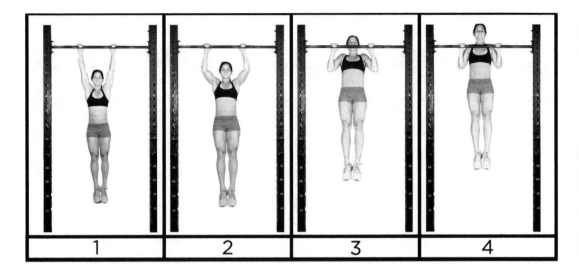

CHIN-UP/PULL-UP MECHANICAL INSTRUCTIONS

1. Squeeze your glutes and position your feet together (or crossed at the ankle if you prefer).
2. Keep your rib cage down to activate abs. Initiate the pull from your lats.
3. Keep your elbows tight and your glutes activated, making sure your lats are your primary movers as you pull yourself toward the bar.
4. Pull your chin up over the bar. Avoid reaching for the bar with your chin. Release with control.

BREATHING INSTRUCTIONS

1. Inhale.
2. Exhale as you pull yourself toward the bar.
3. You may want to hold, then exhale, as you do at any sticking point. Just make sure you don't exhale completely mid-movement.
4. Finish the exhale as your elbows tighten into your body. Inhale as you descend.

NOTE

Did it feel like there was less of an emphasis to your inhale? You are right. The emphasis is on the pull, which makes you more focused on the hold or exhale/hold.

TROUBLESHOOT

Make sure the concept makes sense. On the exhale you are contracting your body; during the chin-up you are contracting your body toward the bar. Visualizing this as an integrated movement rather than an "arm exercise" means you'll get more out of it.

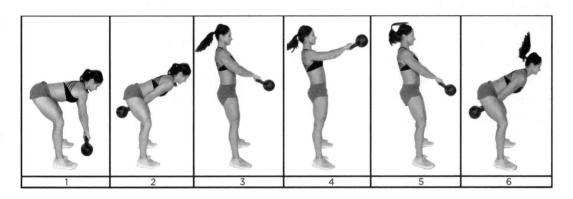

KETTLEBELL SWING MECHANICAL INSTRUCTIONS

1. Keeping your shoulders back, feet slightly wider than hip width, drive your hips back and hinge at the hips with a flat back.
2. As you reach end range, bend your knees and lower your hips—keeping your middle tight and your back flat.
3. Vigorously extend your hips and knees simultaneously. Your arms should not move from the body until your hips reach full extension.
4. Squeeze your glutes as you reach full hip extension. Lock your knees. There will be a moment of weightlessness.
5. Control the kettlebell on the drop.
6. This is the same as the hike of the kettlebell between your legs in step 2, but now with momentum.

BREATHING INSTRUCTIONS

1. Breathe normally as you hinge and prepare.
2. Inhale. Tighten your belly as you transition to projection.
3. Exhale hard. You should be able to hear your exhale.
4. Transition to inhale.
5. Inhale as you backswing.
6. Finish inhale as you are transitioning to projection.

NOTE

While the exhale should be audible and forceful, the inhale may not feel full. Because you have to keep your balance, the inhale should feel as if it's of secondary importance to the exhale, which is giving you power and rhythm. For kettlebells, the transition from the inhale to the exhale to the inhale and the timing of the breath is critical for a perfect movement. You'll also find that with heavier weights and timed reps, you are pushing the weight down, not just letting it "fall."

TROUBLESHOOT

While some coaches will instruct a Reverse Breath (inhale on the way up), be careful. The biggest mistakes when using a Reverse Breath are extending the spine when you should be bracing, and unconsciously moving to a very Vertical Breath, which can unbalance you (especially as you tire).

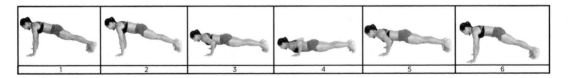

PUSH-UP MECHANICAL INSTRUCTIONS

1. To set up for the push-up, your hands should be slightly wider than your shoulders, fingers turned out.
2. Position yourself so that your shoulders are over your hands, not behind them.

3. As you lower, keep your weight in your hands evenly pressing into the floor.
4. Reach the bottom position. Keep belly tight.
5. As you press out of the bottom position, there should be no change in your spinal or shoulder position. Your back should be flat.
6. Press through your chest, extend your arms, and reestablish the top position.

BREATHING INSTRUCTIONS

1. Breathe normally as you position yourself.
2. Your inhale won't be as audible as your exhale. You might feel some movement at your sides under your armpits.
3. Inhale until your chest touches the floor. Quickly switch to exhale.
4. Exhale hard and enthusiastically.
5. You should feel your ribs move together and narrow slightly.
6. Finish exhale, switch quickly to inhale.

NOTE

Exhale audibly; it will help with pacing and give you a rhythm to follow. The shortened version is: inhale, touch your chest, exhale, press to top.

TROUBLESHOOT

With push-ups you have to maintain a brace while being able to breathe at the same time. Folks who hold their breath will have their form collapse when they finally breathe. If you take big inhales and exhales your brace will fall apart. The best breath for this position is one where the belly stays tight and the sides and back open up slightly. The exhale is not complete; it's just a fast, slight narrow from the inhale.

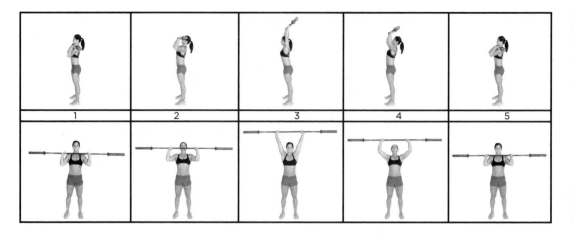

STRICT PRESS MECHANICAL INSTRUCTIONS

1. Establish your stance. The bar is supported by your chest and shoulders. Feet hip-width apart, toes forward. The bar is supported by shoulders (not chest). The bar should travel in a straight line up so you need to lean your head back slightly to get that pretty nose out of the way. Press the bar up, and, once it passes your face, bring your head back in line while looking straight ahead.
2. In one explosive movement, extend your arms.
3. As you lock out your arms overhead, pull your torso and head underneath the bar, maintaining enough tension in your core to balance the bar.
4. As you lower the bar with control, move your nose out of the way.
5. Lower the weight onto your shoulders.

BREATHING INSTRUCTIONS

1. Inhale.
2. Exhale as you extend.
3. Exhale to a brace as you extend your arms. The exhale can be audible.
4. Inhale but with attention, since you are lowering the bar at the same time.
5. As you balance the bar on your body you can take a few small breaths or inhale and go for the next rep.

NOTE

The breathing pattern here relates to load (same as a squat or bench press). With a light weight, it's exhale on the press and inhale on the descent. With a heavy load it's inhale, hold and brace, exhale on the sticking point.

TROUBLESHOOT

Yes, you might feel as if when you are balancing the bar overhead you can sip some air. Just keep it small. Practice high reps at a lower weight, finessing the inhale and transition until it feels perfect.

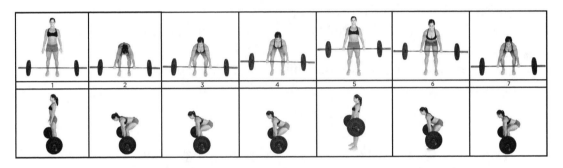

TOP-DOWN SET-UP/DEADLIFT MECHANICAL INSTRUCTIONS

1. Establish your stance, shins at the bar. The bar should bisect the center of your feet.
2. Reach your hamstrings back and hinge at the hips until you can grab the bar or you reach end range.
3. Flatten your back, set your shoulders in a stable position by engaging your lats, and pull your rib cage down to "hug" your body.
4. Sit back slightly as you drive your feet and legs into the floor to pick the bar up.
5. Extend your legs vigorously and straighten to a standing position.
6. If you are doing several reps, reestablish your stance and repeat from step 1.
7. Hinge at the hips to lower the weight to the floor. You may

either gently touch the weight to the floor and rise back up, or put the weight down, reset, and repeat the process.

BREATHING INSTRUCTIONS

1. Inhale and exhale at the bar to focus and prepare.
2. Before the initial lift take an inhale of whatever amount is comfortable for a strong brace.
3. Brace (add a mouthful if you want more pressure).
4. Hold your breath. If you need to exhale slightly at the sticking point, make sure you rebrace to adjust the pressure.
5. Exhale as you bring yourself into a straightened standing position.
6. Inhale and brace as you descend again. (If you are dropping the weight you can take a full breath only once you have let go of the bar.)
7. Add a mouthful of air to your inhale to strengthen your brace here.

NOTE

Depending on the amount of the weight and your strength, you can either exhale halfway up or hold your breath to the top of the rep. The short version: Inhale while standing, hold, brace. Exhale slightly halfway up, rebrace. Hold. Exhale and inhale again.

TROUBLESHOOT

If you start lifting and it doesn't feel right, listen to your gut and stop. Most people will look back and know something didn't feel quite right on that lift that injured them.

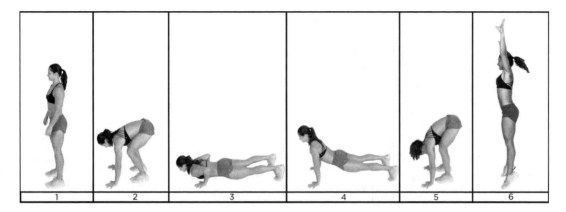

BURPEE MECHANICAL INSTRUCTIONS

1. Beginning stance.
2. Hinge forward at the hips, and place your palms on the ground with your fingers facing straight forward or slightly turned out.
3. Hop your feet back as you lower your chest to the ground.
4. Extend your elbows.
5. Pull your knees toward your chest, hop your feet underneath you (as close to your hands as possible).
6. Drive out of the bottom position into a vertical jump. Absorb your landing and transition into another burpee.

BREATHING INSTRUCTIONS

1. Start inhale as you start to put your hands down.
2. On the second half of your inhale, you are hopping into a plank.
3. Exhale when your chest touches the floor.
4. Start inhale.
5. Exhale as you hop your feet and replace your hands, then short inhale.
6. Exhale as you jump.

NOTE

It's easy for breathing to get chaotic during burpees, especially as you tire. Notice when you switch to mouth breathing, then nasal-bucal on the last few.

TROUBLESHOOT

Because this is fast, focus on the exhales, and the inhales will happen automatically. You may have two exhales or three depending on your fatigue and number of reps.

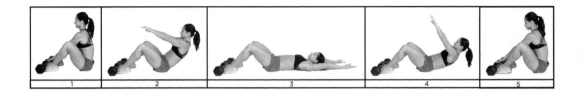

SIT-UP MECHANICAL INSTRUCTIONS

1. Anchor your feet under something (two dumbbells, the couch, a sit-up bench). Start seated; your shoulders are stacked over your hips with your hands touching the dumbbells.
2. Start lowering back.
3. Reach your arms overhead (you can cross them in front of you if you prefer).
4. You may swing your arms as you sit up, reaching in front of you.
5. Come back to your starting position with your shoulders over your hips.

BREATHING INSTRUCTIONS

1. Start your inhale before you start to move. You might feel this as a slight movement of your sides pressing into your legs.
2. Inhale is on the smaller side, so that you can keep your core activated.
3. Finish the inhale as your back touches the floor, and arms extend. Transition to exhale.
4. Exhale as you sit up.
5. Complete the exhale as you come to a seated position.

NOTE

The sound of your breath and the deliberate joining of the breath with the movement can help you get more reps, and more reps of a better quality.

TROUBLESHOOT

Remember that your abdominals and obliques are exhale muscles. If you can get your breathing efficient during this exercise you can recruit more core muscle than you were previously.

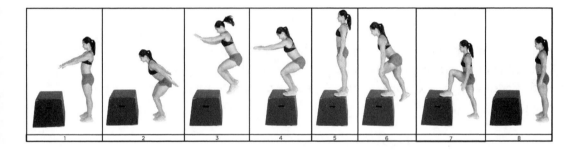

BOX SQUAT MECHANICAL INSTRUCTIONS

1. Start in front of the box with your arms slightly forward of your body.
2. As your arms swing back, hinge at the hips and bend the knees.
3. Quickly swing the arms forward as you explosively jump off the floor.
4. Land on the box as softly as possible.
5. Stand up on the box with your leg muscles engaged.
6. Lean forward slightly as you put one foot back on the ground behind you.
7. Once you've touched the ground, shift your weight and bring the other foot down.
8. Starting position, in front of the box.

BREATHING INSTRUCTIONS

1. Start inhaling.
2. Keep inhaling as you bring your arms back.
3. Exhale as your feet and legs press into the floor to jump.
4. Land as you finish the exhale to help stabilize.
5. Finish the exhale and transition to the inhale.
6. The beginning of this inhale is small, since you will be balancing to bring your foot down.
7. Finish inhale as you bring your other foot down.
8. Exhale at the start position to go again.

NOTE

While intuitively it may feel like when you jump you should inhale, if you are trying to do a set of a movement that needs power and repetition, the exhale is going to be on the push away from the floor.

TROUBLESHOOT

The exhale helps bring your knees up higher. The forceful part of the exhale should not be happening at the landing. If it is, you will be landing too hard. Whether you are stepping down or jumping down or whether you are doing a max height jump will determine whether you take several breaths after the jump or keep with a 1:1 pattern.

FREQUENTLY ASKED QUESTIONS

Q: **What if I am changing the inhale and exhale deliberately because it helps me get more reps with push-ups?**

A: *As long as you don't compromise your posture and your breathing isn't haphazard it's OK. Keep in mind that while you aren't holding weight you have to stay thoughtful and precise about the movement.*

Q: **Should I belly breathe when I have weight on my shoulders?**

A: *No. When you have weight on your body, you are either braced, taking small inhales and exhales by your sides or as needed, or holding*

your breath until the weight is off, when you can take a big decom-
pressive breath. Popping your belly out when you have weight on you
is a one-way ticket to Injuryville.

Q: **When I am squatting with heavier lifts, I am inhaling at the top, holding throughout, then exhaling when I rerack. Is that OK?**

A: *Yes, just make sure that between sets you unbrace and breathe well since you will have spent a fair amount of time with intermittent breath holds as you were lifting.*

Q: **A belly breath feels like it destabilizes me. Is that right?**

A: *Remember a belly breath is just the breath that initiates breathing and that we use to get your probably stuck diaphragm moving. Do not take a belly breath when you are holding a weight. Go back to page 137 and understand the "stiffness spectrum" before you hurt yourself.*

Q: **I actually feel like I want to let air out when I brace deadlifting in step 2. Thoughts?**

A: *If your brace feels solid and safe, then let out a small mouthful. Your brace is not an exhale. In order to get good internal pressure, you have to feel that the entire container that is your body feels solid, and that has to do with both perfect lifting posture and awareness of your own body.*

14

BREATHING FOR PRECISION: LEARNING THE FINE ART OF LETHAL ACCURACY

Displaying precision may be the most satisfying sensation an athlete can experience. It's intoxicating. Whether shooting is for survival or sport, you know that when you hit the target, something feels deeply right. It can be unworldly, almost divine at times. But in fact precision is a skill—one you develop through the intentional practice of eliminating variables. The problem is that, if you are like most athletes, you haven't paid attention to the biggest variable of all: your breathing. In activities where millimeters count, breathing wields a lot of influence—far more than you realize, especially since a detailed, practical discussion of breathing is scant in precision sports literature.

Interestingly, precision for recreational purposes has a long history and deep roots in many cultures. Anthropologists have found depicted what they believe to be a rudimentary form of bowling in an Egyptian tomb that's 3,200 years old. And the game of darts traces its roots back at least to medieval England, where bored soldiers would chuck arrows at the butt end of a cask.

Everyone is trying to find a hack to the infuriating inconsistencies of their game, without homing in on the real problem. The peaks and valleys in performance aren't based on luck, happenstance, flukes, providence, or misfortune. They are moments when your breath is out of sync with your heartbeat and swing, throw, or tap. If your sport or hobby isn't factoring in your breathing, your score is being shaped by variables that you aren't even aware of. For example, every breath you take sets several major muscles and organs on the inside of your body into motion, including the diaphragm, which can move up to five inches from inhalation to exhalation. While this jostle may be imperceptible and seem inconsequential from the outside, it reverberates and affects your access to the bull's-eye.[1]

How you are breathing—or holding your breath—directly affects your nervous system more than anything else you do. More than your "positive self-talk," your therapy sessions addressing your fear of success, or your donning your lucky underwear. Your breathing controls your heart rate, blood pressure, and levels of arousal, anxiety, and adrenaline. Each breath you take sends signals to your brain through the vagus nerve. A less than perfect biomechanical breath speaks to your heart rate and, consequently, affects your jitters.

The pace and depth of your breathing signals your body's autonomic nervous system, which toggles your physical and emotional responses between the extremes of "fight or flight" and "rest and digest." Upper-chest breathing makes your body think you are under attack and it responds in time, pumping more cortisol and adrenaline into your system (which may be only one teaspoon, but if your goal is to be precise, that is one teaspoon too much). That's helpful when you're trying to outrun a bear (or in a huddle and being psyched up by your football coach), but counterproductive when your goal is to sink a pool shot or hit your mark. Modern life pushes us to extremes, and in precision sports your success depends on your being able to stay squarely in a perfectly calibrated calm and alert state, with sophisticated fine motor skills—a place foreign to most other sports.

PRINCIPLES OF PRECISION

The principles of breathing for precision that you should integrate into your understanding will:

1. Lower your body's center of gravity, allowing you to gain better stability.
2. Minimize unmitigated upper-body movement.

---

1   The USMC Instructor Guide specifies that shots be timed to the natural respiratory pause or the moment after an exhale when muscles and movement calm down and "the scope has settled."

3. Control your nervous system in order to avert anxiety and channel that energy into improved performance.

4. Lower your heart rate and blood pressure at will, reining in stress hormones such as cortisol.

5. Efficiently oxygenate your body and brain to give you consistent clarity and calm.

6. Tune in to your intuition and turn off mental chatter.

7. Maintain focus and attention throughout long performances.

BREATHING EXERCISES: THE MENTAL LINK BETWEEN THE GAME AND THE MECHANICS

Just as you should crawl before you walk and walk before you run, the techniques for developing precision are best learned through baby steps. You'll learn the fundamental steps to take for accuracy and consistency through a combination of examples of two sport situations that are highly controllable: putting in golf and shooting at a target range. These are two models of precision sports in which there are fewer variables: the target isn't moving, you aren't moving, and you aren't in a crowded arena full of people noisily encouraging you or shouting insults. What you learn is applicable to other precision sports such as archery, darts, billiards, knives, or axe throwing.[2]

Here is a very boiled-down list of some of the best takeaways from research related to precision. (All the references are in the footnotes or in the bibliography for those of you who want to go back to the original studies.)

> Not all precision sports are alike. But breathing is critical for performance in all of them. In archery, your arm position is strikingly different from the one you use in golf. In billiards, you are leaned over; in holding a bow, you are sliding your fingers back to shoot; with a gun, you are pressing the trigger; and in golf, you tap the ball.

1. The biggest threat to precision is eye and head movement.

2. Our attention spans are getting shorter; hence, your ability to be precise is directly related to your ability to pay attention.

---

2   A lesser known precision sport is conger cuddling in the UK, where a dead eel is thrown at members of the Royal National Lifeboat Institution. The sport was banned in 2006.

3. What you repeat to yourself doesn't matter as much as you think.

4. Your ability to lower your heart rate is critical.

5. Tension creates jerky movements. Fluidity means that you aren't only thinking calm thoughts, but your body is calm as well.

6. Your choice of inhale or exhale before choosing your "go time" is crucial to success.

7. Fine motor control goes out the window when you cross the threshold from alert to anxious.

8. Anxiety warps your sense of time and your auditory input. Outside distractors—from that chirping bird to that whispering at the periphery—can sound much louder than they are.

9. Hypoxia sets in. What does low oxygen—hypoxia—feel like? It's decreased attention, poor judgment, loss of motor skills and coordination.

10. In a high-stakes situation, your heart rate rises (regardless of how much precision the situation needs). And what you are telling yourself ("It's just a game, relax!") is often a lie, about which we'll talk soon. The stakes don't need to be "real"; they just need to matter to you.

11. Intermittent breath holding can negatively affect your performance.

12. CO_2 buildup creates an urgency to breathe that is detrimental to your ability to aim. Discomfort with CO_2 buildup and anxiety over feelings of breathlessness are well documented.

13. Your sights will inevitably drift slightly upward on an inhale, and downward during an exhale. A Vertical Breath will exacerbate that.

14. "Slow play"—taking too much time and becoming overwhelmed with mechanics—is the foe of precision athletes.

A study at Griffith University in Australia that appeared in the *International Journal of Psychophysiology* examined the heart rates and breathing patterns when golfers of varying abilities putted, and found that the more experienced and elite golfers "showed a pronounced phasic deceleration in heart rate immediately prior to the putt [and] greater heart rate variability in the very low frequency band." Translation: They came in to the putt with a lower heart rate, and were able to slow it down even more prior to the putt itself. The study authors noticed something else interesting: The more skilled golfers also exhaled just before putting, which makes sense, since exhalations slow down your heart. The novice golfers, on the other hand, tended to inhale before moving their club.

IT'S NOT YOUR IMAGINATION.
YOUR HEART REALLY IS RACING IN
HIGH-STAKES SITUATIONS

Focus and fine motor skills are two of the abilities that are affected by an adrenaline dump or feelings of anxiety.[3] While you may be able to take long steps and swing your arms, threading a needle becomes very difficult.[4] As you cross the line from alert to anxious, blood will be drawn away from your extremities. As the game progresses, the pressure builds and your ability to relax becomes key. Fluidity and consistency suffer.

FREQUENTLY ASKED QUESTIONS

Q: **People say thinking about breathing will just add more complexity to the huge list of mechanics I already have. Will it?**

A: *Your breathing is not part of your mechanics. In fact, focusing on your inhale and exhale will distract you from obsessing on your mechanics. Which is why the Targeted Breathing Model we'll talk about in the next chapter shows that when it comes time to execute, you aren't giving conscious thought to your breath. You can pay attention to your breathing at every other stage, from when you arrive and do a*

---

3   In one of the more intrusive examinations of golfing and breathing, scientists at Rutgers University outfitted a visor with infrared sensors for tracking breathing and heart rate, and two others that recorded head movement and eye movement. They placed the headgear onto six participants (all of them novices at golf), had them hit 20 putts from 9 feet away. At first, participants would receive 2 points for each putt made, and lose 2 for every putt they missed. Then researchers upped the pressure, assigning bigger and bigger penalties (up to 5 points) to the misses. The results, published in the *Journal of Strength and Conditioning Research*, recorded that as the stakes grew higher, the golfers' heartbeats raced faster, pumping about 10 more beats per minute than they did in the early (less penalized) rounds.

4   And as first responders will tell you, the next things affected are auditory perception, sense of time, and memory. For ongoing fascinating research on memory follow Dr. Janet Metcalfe's work at Columbia University's Metacognition and Memory Lab at http://www.columbia.edu/cu/psychology/metcalfe/index.html

warm-up to when you perform your pre-shot routine. And that's where the ability of the breath to distract you is actually a good thing. By focusing in on your breath during your pre-shot, you can use it to stop the chatter going on inside your mind. When your mind is quiet, you are fully present. When you are fully present, you are in flow. And when you are in flow, you perform your best.

BETTER STABILITY FROM WHICH TO SHOOT

Do you know where your center of gravity is, really? Well, it's not where you think it is. In order to understand why, let's clear up some misconceptions about the core. When people are asked where their core is, they will point to a space roughly a few inches above their belly button. Or they'll make a circular motion around the middle of their torso. In reality, you have to move the location down, way down, about half a foot. Your pelvis, abdominals, obliques, and back are your core, along with the twenty or so muscles that make up your pelvic floor and support everything above it. Your core doesn't just wrap around your middle, it wraps around the bottom of your torso, too. So now let's reorient your body to this new information. Your center of gravity refers to the space two inches under your belly button, right where your belt is. That is your anchor, your anatomical middle. If you breathe and let your middle expand and contract there, you are automatically going to have a lower center of gravity, which, in the long run, will give you a stronger drive and better base.[5]

Whatever your precision game is, it's always about numbers and physics. Later we will cover the "inner game" that supports your mechanics—and it's not about self-talk, vision, or divine intervention. If you aren't tapping into your internal game and flow/tempo, you are going to have to deal with ups and downs in performance that will make you want to throw in the towel.

Dr. Richard Coop, a golf psychologist with more than forty years of experience coaching Division I athletes and professional golfers—including a young Michael Jordan—tagged the concept of a "cleansing breath," or a breath where you inhale through the nose then exhale through the mouth.

---

5   Check out talks by Taoist Master Mantak Chia, who explains why the gut and this space around your belly button are essential for physical, emotional health, and energy (as per Taoist tradition).

CASE STUDY

From Belisa: Mark was a big man with a big chest. His initial Vertical Breath moved the entire top of his body up visibly with every breath. He had constant neck and shoulder pain (and TMJ). First, I moved his breath down to his middle and belly so that his shoulders could relax and he'd feel as if he had a better breath. His sensation of not getting enough air (which was puzzling to him because of his large rib cage) had to do with not exhaling well—not emptying out fully. The weight he carried on his belly made exhaling more difficult; as a result, he had taken on the bad habit of barely exhaling.

Mark thought the "air hunger" he was feeling was a result of trying to focus and be still. When he would pause to try to take a deep breath, his whole body would jostle upward. The concept of "over-inflating" is particularly relevant to dysfunctional Vertical Breathers. Unfortunately, the response was to just take a really small breath. Given that Mark was probably already "hovering"—taking tiny breaths out of bad habit—the end result was tension and disrupted CO_2/O_2.

When Mark learned to breathe horizontally, he was able to take breaths that felt as if they were at 80 percent, and were exponentially better than upper-body breaths in terms of quantity of air. He set an imaginary line below his pecs and brought attention to everything underneath moving on the inhale. Breathing with the hip tilt and understanding the mechanics solidified the change. The result was less unmitigated upper-body movements, less low-grade anxiety because of feelings of "not getting enough air," and, ultimately, better scores.

PGA Championship winner Jason Dufner used a strategy borrowed from Marine snipers to get his putting under control. "There's been times with my putting that the thought process and my actions have felt like they've been sped up and too quick," Dufner told *USA Today*. "I'm trying to slow down and focus on that breathing. It's been working." As of late 2018, Phil Mickelson was the most accurate putter on the PGA Tour. Just before Mickelson sunk a par-3 playoff putt to win the 2013 PGA, National Teacher of the Year, Lou Guzzi said, "You could see how focused he was on his breathing, taking in oxygen and getting himself as relaxed as possible before playing the shot." And 2013 U.S. Open champion Justin Rose says, "After three deep breaths, it's amazing how much calmer you'll feel." As with most breathing advice in golf, it doesn't go into specifics, but we do.

For your swing, look to see what your body finds natural, and then practice it consciously. It is not another mechanic

> *that you have to check off as the seconds tick on the green. You should know exactly how many breaths you take to the ball and what your breath looks like at the ball. On the swing, exhale on effort.*

BEFORE GOING ON, EVALUATE YOURSELF: RPM (RESPIRATORY PRECISION METRICS)

These are the numbers you need to have as your baselines:

What is your resting heart rate?	
What is your best inhale hold time?	
What is your best exhale hold time?	
How low can you bring down your heart rate?	
At what HR is your sweet spot/natural pause?	
What is your Breathing IQ (your LOM and ROM)?	

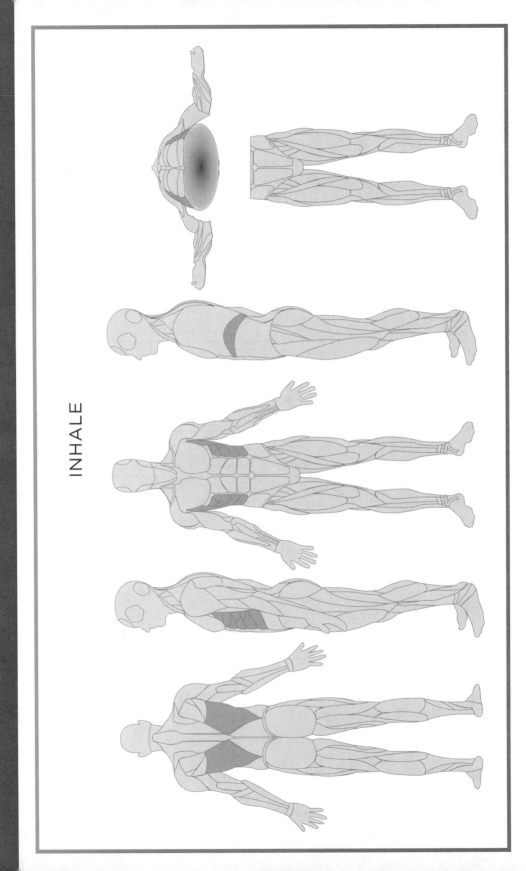

GOOD BREATHING INHALE

INHALE

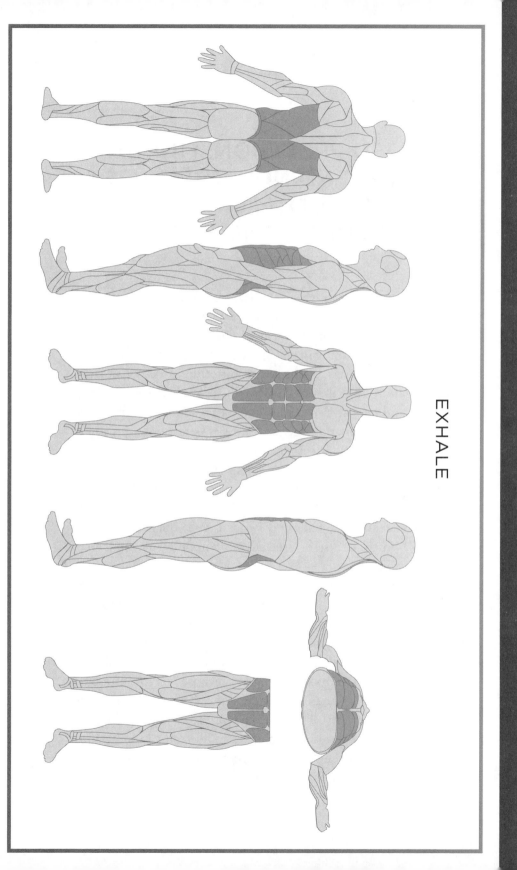

EXHALE

GOOD BREATHING EXHALE

15

APPLIED PRECISION: FINDING (AND EXTENDING) "THE SWEET SPOT" IN GOLF, SHOOTING, ARCHERY, AND POOL

Here's another story from Belisa's teachings: When I first examined the breathing of many of the golfers I worked with, I was surprised to find . . . well, that there wasn't any. "There's no crying in baseball, and apparently no breathing in golf, either," I would joke with them.

Indeed, the majority of the precision athletes do what I call "hover," meaning that they take a small sip of air in, hold briefly, then exhale and repeat. It's a natural human response to stress, and if you want to control and override your stress response, it's something you have to dismantle and study.

And sure, it seems to make sense that if you are tunnel-vision-level focused on something bull's-eye-like, you should do what any animal would do: make the smallest movements possible, including your breathing. That's why I equate it to "the modern predatory state" (which we also can see at your computer, as you lean in to meet a deadline).

Part of the reason for quiet breathing on the course is driven by the culture of the sport. Professional billiards matches and golf games are notoriously quiet places. So, you become a notoriously quiet breather. Even celebrations that allow for a fist pump are almost always virtually silent. You wouldn't dare let loose with that *yes!* you know you want to shout (in part because you are supposed to have nerves of steel and unflinching confidence. Of course, you were going to win, right?). The reverse is also true. When things go wrong, you can't go shouting expletives. The result is something akin to "repressed adrenaline" or unmetabolized tension. (Don't worry; instructions on what to do about this are forthcoming.)

DO THIS NOW

Watch an animal shift gears. They "shake it off." As humans we are terrible at finding an equivalent to letting the steam out of the kettle. And instructions to "let it go" are cerebral; they are not read by your nervous system. When this predatory state turns primal and hijacks your prefrontal cortex, mayhem ensues, which, justified or not, includes the throwing of helmets.[1]

The following principles and exercises are for any game that requires precision. They are, in fact, the three pillars upon which rest breathing and precision sports. Make sure you agree with the following:

1. Breathing between shots is critical. Between shots, breathing in an anatomically congruent manner loosens my body, which keeps me calm but alert and oxygenates my muscles and brain.
2. How precisely I integrate my breathing into my pre-shot routine is decisive. Breathing keeps me from dwelling on the mechanics; it's not another mechanic. Focusing on my breathing means that I can let my body tap into what it knows and has practiced without my brain interrupting.
3. Breathing horizontally is vital because it keeps unmitigated movements at bay. Any movements that I make are deliberate and practiced; nothing is left to chance.

The exercises you are learning create the foundation on which you will develop these three critical pieces of the game. In this chapter I'm going to ask for you to draw up a targeted breathing plan, which is much like a map of your breathing and movements.

---

1   By Brett Lawrie, Brandon Jacobs, and Mike Shildt; Gatorade jugs (Mark Cuban); punching objects like fire extinguishers (Amare Stoudemier), clubhouse doors (AJ Burnette); or make for post-fight tussles such as in Khabib Nurmagomedov and Conor McGregor's UFC 229 fight.

FINDING THE "NATURAL RESPIRATORY PAUSE"

When shooting a gun, the natural respiratory pause comes after "the scope settles," meaning that the jiggle inside your field of vision has stopped. You do this by stilling your body and breath. Recognize that there is a difference between holding your breath to try to find it and finding the natural pause on the exhale. Know your pre-shot routine, "find the natural pause," and practice it. Right now, you can recognize the reverse: you take the shot and it feels "wrong."

> *Sweet spot is about optimum pressure in archery. But you also have a sweet spot in your timing. Here is where your attention to detail that is part of your love of your precision sport comes into play.*

Knowing when in the breathing spectrum you let go, pull the trigger, and take the shot is essential because you can't be consistent if you can't recognize the moment and conjure it repeatedly. If that moment of natural respiratory pause isn't something you can identify 100 percent of the time, you are leaving part of your game up to chance.

You want to be able to access that moment at will, and make it replicable. Every. Single. Time.

GOLF IS LIKE SHOOTING,
BUT SHOOTING IS NOT LIKE GOLF

The U.S. Marines rifle training guide instructs shooters to breathe, aim during the exhale, breathe again, exhale again, and then fire during what they call the "natural respiratory pause," or the moment when your heart is beating the slowest and therefore your hand is at its most steady. The exhale also releases tension in your outer intercostal muscles.

The "natural respiratory pause" or "sweet spot" is not just holding your breath. A breath hold can happen anywhere during the breath cycle, but the natural respiratory pause occurs *after an exhale*. In fact, pausing on an inhale is known to be less accurate owing to

Some experts may recommend shooting "on the exhale" or "at the bottom of the exhale." This good advice turns bad because the foundation—the mechanics of the inhale and exhale—are wrong. A Vertical Breath will always be shallower; a Horizontal Breath will always lower your heart rate best. Note the cues that encourage a dysfunctional Vertical Breath, like the "bottom" of an exhale. In a vertical exhale, the time you exhale will be shorter and the red light in your body that signals you are "out of air" will come on much faster.

the fact that when you pause on an inhale in shooting, air leakage will inevitably occur from the nose or mouth, so your sights will drift. Furthermore, from a physiological perspective, the natural respiratory pause occurs with a slowing down of the heart. If you were to hook up an EKG to an expert marksman, you would actually see the heart decelerate. You'll also notice that the deceleration occurs for several seconds, so the "pause" isn't just a blip. The natural respiratory pause should feel exactly as its name indicates: *natural*. You'll almost feel as if you don't have to inhale. At first many struggle to find the natural respiratory pause. They are so externally focused that going inward and tuning in to the heart can be a challenge.

ADJUST YOUR PRE-SHOT

You drop yourself into your zone with both the first step and first breath you take, which gives you access to flow/tempo. Your shot doesn't start when you step up—it starts once you've made an assessment and move to strike and take your first step. The top players in precision sports do this automatically. How many breaths to the target? Your breath should move with you. Not tag along haphazardly. Right now, map out your pre-shot routine and add your breath. At no point should you not know whether you are in an inhale or exhale.

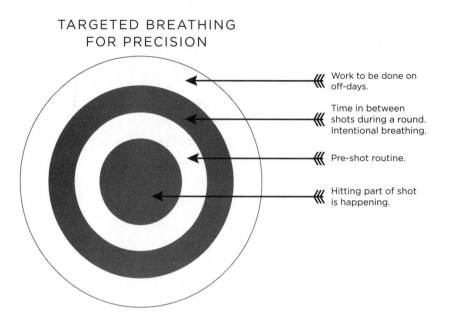

TARGETED BREATHING
FOR PRECISION

Work to be done on off-days.

Time in between shots during a round. Intentional breathing.

Pre-shot routine.

Hitting part of shot is happening.

POINTS FOR TARGETED BREATHING FOR PRECISION

- The bull's-eye is the moment when you shoot—whether it's a dart, hatchet, marble, or 9mm. The "thinking part" of your shot is over, and the "hitting part" is happening.

- The first circle is your pre-shot routine. When driving or chipping, you choose your target. During a putt, you read the greens, maybe, and plumb bob. But then there's a point at which you bring that pre-shot thinking and analysis to an end. There's an old saying in golf: "The thinking must stop before the hitting begins." Your breathing can provide the break. You physically decide to turn off your brain and focus first on your breathing, and then on the execution.

- The second circle encompasses all the time between each shot you take during a round. It's a time best spent keeping your body and mind relaxed. You'll see golfers employ all kinds of techniques in order to do this. This is the time when you can use intentional breathing to keep your body and mind right.

- The third circle out indicates the work you should be doing on off-days. Spoiler alert: it involves stretching. Rotation places a lot of demands on your torso.

YES, BODY TYPE MATTERS

I f you are on the heavy side, you'll have to work on your exhale. If you are very thin, you'll find you are in an "exhale" all the time. Letting your middle expand for a good inhale takes some work. In both cases you are using different muscles, muscles that need training.

> "Many golfers unknowingly hold their breath, or take quick shallow breaths when hitting difficult shots or stroking important putts," Dr. Deborah Graham points out in her book, *The 8 Traits of Champion Golfers: How to Develop the Mental Game of a Pro.*

Using your primary breathing muscles as we are coaching you to do now instead of your auxiliary muscles as you usually do will mean a complete reorganization of your game. As a consequence, you will be able to get out of a plateau and really control your nervous system.

DO THIS NOW

Do it wrong (for the last time), then do it right. Lean over the pool table or hinge over the golf ball. Take a "bad" Vertical Breath. Do this in an exaggerated way to understand the subtlety of what happens. Stand over the ball and take a Horizontal Breath. Notice the difference. These are the details that make a tremendous difference in precision sports.

Precision sports depend on the consistency of nuance.

FIND THE "SWEET SPOT" IN YOUR BREATH (AND HOW TO CONJURE IT MORE CONSISTENTLY)

O nce you have that long inhale and exhale (the B-IQ grade of an "A"), start seeing where in your body you can feel your pulse. Close your eyes now and see if you can feel it. Is it an almost inaudible pulsating inside your ears, a feeling in your fingers or lips? Or can you feel a patterned movement in your chest? The more optimal inhale and longer length of exhale time you have means very concretely that your heart rate will lower and that "perfect timing" will become more and more apparent. What this is physiologically is that you are getting to sense your heart rate.

TECHNIQUES FOR REFINING YOUR BREATHING

Slowing or "lengthening" the exhale is hard. Most people have a hard time for two reasons:

1. Their inhale is mediocre, so lengthening the exhale is hard because they "run out of air."
2. Lengthening the exhale is hard because it is an isometric muscular exercise. If you don't control it, those small but important muscles are weak.

-   Once you start breathing horizontally you'll simply be taking a better, more efficient, bigger breath. There is no magic here: your exhale will be longer because you have more air.
-   Your exhale will get longer because you will empty out better. You now understand that the exhale should be narrow, which is significantly different than a vertical exhale where you just let go.
-   Want proof? Time your exhale. Once you have gotten to an "A" B-IQ score (wide inhale, narrow exhale, and no shoulder movement) your exhale will change significantly. Immediately.

DO THIS NOW

The next big inhale starts at your hips. You may put your hand at your hip or pocket to facilitate this. The movement is slight, but your tailbone tips out (anterior pelvic tilt) on the inhale, and under (posterior) on the exhale. You pay attention to your center, two inches under your belly button. As you inhale and exhale, your attention goes here (not to your head, face, and upper chest the way it did before). You bring attention to your feet and feel connected to the ground, a concept that finally makes sense kinesthetically because your breath isn't up by your collarbones. The combination of these things lowers your heart rate, lowers your blood pressure, and kicks in your parasympathetic nervous system. Your pelvis—the powerhouse—feels strong. Your arms and shoulders now can feel like what they are: a flexible pendulum for your upper body.[2]

---

2   You keep a lower breath, but go to 50 percent so that there is no chance of "overinflating." It is really just the bottom of your body.

THE PRE-SHOT ROUTINE

Say your competitor finishes their pool shots and all eyes turn to you. Typically, your shot would have started as you pick your position in back of the pool ball. Wrong—this is way too late. Rewind five seconds . . . However many steps you take or practice shots you make (if any), have them be coordinated with the breath. At first, this was work pairing them; now it is almost subconscious. Movement, intention, and your own internal tempo working together.[3]

When you use your diaphragm to breathe horizontally, you are more stable; you are breathing in a way that lowers your center of gravity and frees up your body to be calmer and more flexible. When you use your diaphragm to breathe horizontally your breath will be "bigger" (up to six times the amount of a Vertical Breath) and your natural pause is going to be longer. That moment will be stretched out so eventually you can recognize it more clearly. The stability of your body and the clarity of your natural pause depend on whether your breath is biomechanically sound. If that is the case, you will find that:

- You are automatically calmer, clearer.
- Your body is looser, less tense.
- Your center of gravity is low; it's the best center of balance you can have.
- Your breathing feels like it is fueling you because now it is.
- Essentially you are syncing up the inside of your body, so your muscles, brain, and training do what you want "on the outside."

PREDATOR BREATHING:
UPREGULATING AND DOWNREGULATING

Many sports require the ability to charge up, then charge down, and quieten and conserve energy. Think hockey or hatchet

---

3   Dr. Gregg Steinberg, a sports psychologist who comments on PGATour.com, says that any good pre-shot routine starts with a breath.

throwing: you want to have flexibility in your focus and energy level. Precision sports require you to be "on" and "off." You need to be upregulating to be alert and focused, and downregulating in order to keep calm between shots (and not let the previous or future shot affect you). You don't want to stay stone-faced and calm throughout; inside you want your body to go from focused and still to recover, then unwind over and over again.

The hardest thing to do is what SWAT snipers and biathlon athletes do: move quickly during an emergency, then, with unfailing precision, fire accurately. It is so challenging because simple range training doesn't translate to these situations. Often we use the technique they do: freezing and settling (which is easier if you've been heel-toeing into a room rather than barging through a door). At times we don't have to, at times we should be finding the natural pause. If you are in a sport that has the luxury of a few seconds for you to find that sweet spot to let go of the arrow, putt, or shot, practice it.

While few people will list race car driving as a precision sport, it most certainly is. It is a unique hybrid of endurance and precision. Take g-force, heat, fumes, noise, the intense tremor of the car, and weight of the wheel, and add the limiting posture of the seat that restricts breathing and the need for your attention and vision to be critically accurate. It has an element of chase, pounce, chase, pounce as the driver whips around corners. The requirement of precision plus endurance is built in, and the element of danger keeps the driver focused. Sports that are dangerous hold your attention by the urgency of the situation.

HOW DO I PRACTICE THIS?

- *Inhale and feel your entire body expand.* This is the breath that brings blood to all your extremities. Look off into the distance, exhale slowly, feel your heart rate slow, feel that your center of gravity is low. The idea of a low, efficient, circumferential abdominothoracic breath is not a vague notion. You should have numbers and body cues to guide you. Same with your heart rate: you should be able to guess it within a narrow range and precise numbers.

- *Move into focus.* As your focus narrows, so does your breath. They go hand in hand. Practice widening your field of vision and widening your breath, then narrowing your field of vision and narrowing your breath. You feel the breath at your nostrils; it's more contained now. Your vision focuses to your task. Your lips are together but your jaw is slack. The sensation of this focused breath of yours is your focus.
- *You position yourself.* Then on the next exhale, recognize the pause.

TIMING THE SETTLE

Whether you are walking over to throw a hatchet or bending over a pool table, your body needs to settle. You need one extra breath to have your muscles go from movement to stillness. If you breathe badly, this never seems like enough time. However, once you change your breathing to a more perfect breath, one breath is more than enough to align yourself to then look for the exhale natural pause.

And keep in mind that when you run, your diaphragm is the muscle that helps you go from movement to still. It is the center plate in your body that brings things to a halt, and you also need it to inhale and exhale. Recognizing how your breath changes in response to movement—locomotive pairing—is what distinguishes between good and great.

EXERCISE

1. Take five fast steps.
2. Hit your timer/watch.
3. Close your eyes; find that natural pause.
4. Look at the number.
5. Do this 100 times.
6. Now make it 10 steps, same drill.
7. Advanced: add distractors.

WHY IS THIS SO HARD?

Exhaling slowly to find the natural pause when you are a Vertical Breather is excruciating. Why? You did it to yourself. A Vertical Breath is going to be shorter so the moment of pause will be tiny, sometimes imperceptible. Trying to find that blip on the screen when the screen is so narrow makes your job challenging. What to do? Extend the exhale. The practice of sensing the natural pause happens more often, so even if breath gets shallow for a few seconds, while you are over the ball again you can find it.

EXTEND YOUR EXHALE

Time your exhale. Inhale a full breath, without moving your shoulders. Hit the timer and start exhaling. Note the numbers where you go from comfortable exhale to slightly more attentive, then uncomfortable, then really uncomfortable. Note your total number.

These numbers are going to be very different, and they should be. And you should be sensitive to the difference between them and how they change.

As your B-IQ gets closer to an "A" and you learn to pace your breath so that you are using muscles that have to do with slowing the exhale, this will change.

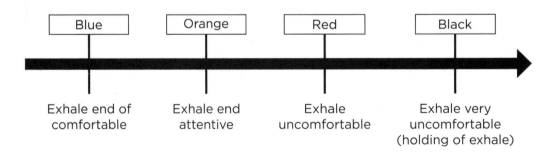

YOUR STORIES

"When I first did this exercise, I had just started changing my breathing, so I was a "C" B-IQ. I know I should have practiced to get to an "A," then moved to the precision chapter, but I went ahead anyway. When I was a "C" my exhale blue was 10, orange was 12, red was 16, and black was 26. Once I got my B-IQ to an "A," I felt like I had more air to exhale and all my numbers went up about ten seconds. I got really diligent and kept a notebook. What I noticed is that I was more comfortable 'in an exhale' than I had ever been before. I could pinpoint the second when I felt really stable better than I ever could before."

—*Mark B.*

"When I recalculated my shot as starting after my visual assessment of the situation, and my starting to move to the shot, several things happened: the time I was shooting started sooner, and there wasn't the spike in anxiety right when I was supposed to shoot. The breathing with every step made me immediately feel under control before striking, and made it feel familiar so that I could relax into what I was familiar with."

—*Morgan F.*

"Focusing on my breathing meant I wasn't distracted by sounds on the periphery or the chatter in my head. I practiced this during the day—I'd guess five steps to the door from my desk. I'd take the steps with the breath, and it made for an 'on-ramp' that smoothed out and sped up my performance."

—*Michael B.*

"I had plateaued as far as my performance in archery. Then, I added very deliberate breathing exercises. I started by backing up and noticing the way I breathed in excruciating detail. First thing I noticed is that I didn't have an exact pattern. I would just 'steady' my breath. Now, I start by making sure I am taking a low horizontal breath, I relax, and keep my gaze and jaw soft. I get into stance, grip, put my arrow on the bow, and draw and align with the target all in the same number of breaths each time. Plus now I get into my stance really being oxygenated and relaxed whereas before I just vacillated on different levels of tense. As soon as I let go of the arrow, the next breath immediately is wide and low. My whole game is now connected and feels more fluid."

—Liah J.

> It's not so much what you are doing at the shot; it is the mechanics you have practiced. It's more about changing the breath to be one that is anatomically congruous, being consistent with your breathing and rebooting between shots so you aren't tapping into your energy when you don't need to.

ADVANCED EXERCISE:
LISTEN TO YOUR HEART

What you are gaining access to is the ability to sense your heart rate, and rather than guessing or hoping it doesn't interfere, you are using it to your advantage.

An advanced exercise, once you have that long inhale and exhale down, is to start seeing where in your body you can feel your pulse. Close your eyes now and see if you can feel it. Is it an almost inaudible pulsating inside your ears, a feeling in your fingers or lips? Practice feeling your heart rate. Vary the amount of noise around you. See if you can sense it even when you are angry or irritated. Once you can feel it, see if you can guess it (10 seconds x 6) and with an HR monitor see how close you are. Change the setting to more or less loud, more or less emotional, and guess.

In what other two situations do you have to work on extending the exhale? If you are a free diver or if you are presenting on stage and need to make it to the end of a sentence. In both cases, you also have to tolerate holding your breath on the exhale. The exhale is a controlled one that gives you time. While these don't require precision, they do require the same attention to an extended exhale.

DO THIS NOW

Two seldom-considered exercises that help your golf game:

1. Kettlebells help the golf game in an unorthodox way, by bringing the breath back to the swing: you are "allowed to exhale" and hear your breath (whereas in golf, grunts are outlawed). The swing of the kettlebell must be paired with the breath. Even light kettlebells help you relearn to integrate the breath and movement again.

2. Deadlifting with a large side of grunt. While you don't have the ticking of the clock, you are keenly aware of time. Taking too much time between shots? Powerlifting stops the dawdle. You never see powerlifters pondering over the bar. They walk over, move it, walk away. That flow is what is missing in golf. You give yourself too much time to think and hence get in your own way. Even if you practice with less than a powerlifting load, try it, and take some pointers from powerlifters. Golf like a powerlifter.[4]

OTHER SPORTS THAT NEED EXTENDED EXHALES

BET (FOR FREE DIVING)

Breathe: Make sure your lung capacity is maximal (use spirometry, FVC to measure this).
Extend: Your exhale. You are using very different muscles than your inhale, different muscles than when you do quick Exhale Pulsations. This is really almost an isometric exercise.
Tolerate: Discomfort. Whether it's rising CO_2 or the weight of the water above you, practicing discomfort will help it change from painful to annoying. Next step is to relax.

THE BEAUTIFUL TRIFECTA

When breathing horizontally, the trifecta of lungs, heart, and diaphragm form an exquisite pulsating triangle in which each component supports the other. Why aren't we taught how these organs move together? If you learn anything from this book, it's that there should be a symphony of coordinated movement inside your body, with your lungs and diaphragm massaging your heart. And below, your digestive organs and pelvic floor are affected by the thoracic diaphragm's engagement. Without this very natural inner movement,

---

4   Dr. Lucius Riccio's number-one rule for individuals is that you need to always walk directly to your own ball at a speed of three miles per hour or more. His book, *Golf's Pace of Play Bible*, has earned him the title "Pope of Pace."

it's more a cacophony than a symphony, and we become toxic and anxious. Maybe you've had a fleeting moment experiencing the congruence of all three: when you see them working together in your mind's eye, and then almost feel as if you are "in the zone" for a few seconds. In the beginning, the disjointedness or numbness of this process will be what is noticeable. Be assured that that zone-like feeling is replicable.

16

BREATHING FOR RECOVERY: TECHNIQUES TO COME BACK FASTER AND STRONGER

What first comes to mind when most people think about recovery? Perhaps leaning back, putting your feet up, and resting on "the seventh day." Or maybe the seasons when fields lie fallow, or adding more yin to your yang. However, for warriors, *recovery* refers to achieving a balance that lies between activity and inactivity, movement and sedentariness, exertion and repose.

It used to be that *recovery* meant taking a day off or even enjoying a "cheat day," but things have changed. The newest sport science is telling us the same thing: the key to longevity in any sport isn't being the biggest, fastest, or strongest. The true secret is being able to recover between performances, because recovery is the time your muscles grow and information gets integrated in your brain.

Recently the word *regeneration* has been heard alongside *recovery*. But the concept is not new. At Hippolyte Triat's gym in Paris, which is widely regarded as the world's first commercial gym, the sign above the door at the gym reads, THE REGENERATION OF MAN.[1] And Mark Verstegen, founder of EXOS and director of performance for the NFL Players Association, has popularized the idea of "regeneration days" in his insightful book, *Core Performance: The Revolutionary Workout Program to Transform Your Body and Your Life*.

---

1   An interesting note, related by Eric Chaline, in *The Temple of Perfection: A History of the Gym*.

WORK HARD, RECOVER HARD:
ACTIVE RECOVERY

Active recovery may sound like an oxymoron, but perhaps the most interesting turn of fortune in recent years is how recovery has gone from "just resting" to something you do with intention and planning. The need to be at the top of your game "on demand" now means recovery times have to be effective and even measurable as far as their results are concerned.

The concept of *active recovery* is winning fans in the strength and conditioning world for many reasons:

1. Research shows that fairly intense exercise (at or above 60 percent of your heart rate max) can increase cortisol. However, a study published in the *Journal of Endocrinological Investigations* in 2008 pointed out that exercise at a more relaxed effort (40 percent of heart rate max or below) can decrease baseline cortisol levels, which means that an easy workout can actually reduce stress chemicals in your body.

2. A study out of Poland led by Anna Mika examined twelve soccer players and thirteen mountain canoeists and found that they recovered faster and felt less leg fatigue when they performed twenty minutes of active recovery after workouts.

3. Multiple studies[3] indicate that active recovery can lower lactate concentrations within the body, indicating that athletes were better able to perform in subsequent workouts.

> "More effort works…but not when it comes to recovery," says Coach Ingrid "The Iron Valkyrie" Marcum. "A sympathetically driven athlete probably hasn't been in a parasympathetic state for a while. High achievers know a lot of information, but most success comes with effort, with force, and with recovery, this isn't the case. The relaxation that you need to drop into a state is the exact opposite of what you are used to. And we need that if we want to really recover and go hard again."[2]

---

2   Interview on April 2, 2019. Marcum is a multisport athlete and strength and conditioning coach. Her five-part series on breathing can be found at http://www.ingridmarcum.com/breathing-for-performance.

3   For example: Lopes, Felipe A. S. et al. "The effect of active recovery on power performance during the bench press exercise." *Journal of Human Kinetics*; Draper, Nick et al. "Effects of Active Recovery on Lactate Concentration, Heart Rate and RPE in Climbing." *Journal of Sports Science & Medicine.*

ADD A LITTLE PSYCH TO THE
RECOVERY PROCESS

Adding a psychological component is essential to recovery: Have you internalized your dad's screaming at you that you aren't ever going to amount to anything to such a point that still decades later you are trying to prove him wrong, to the point of injury? Is there still a version of an eight-year-old self in your thirty-five-year-old body trying to please a parent, fit into the team, be stronger than a bully? These are the self-imposed obstacles that get in the way of your respecting your intuition, and perhaps not allowing yourself that healing extra half hour of sleep.

> *"If you are a person who is evolving in terms of their personal development, you have to add components of emotional and interpersonal challenges to your personal curriculum," says strength and performance expert Jason Ferruggia. ". . . Talk about fear, vulnerability, relationships in addition to lifting heavy and hard."*[4]

NEW DEVELOPMENTS IN RECOVERY
HAVE DEEP ROOTS

While cold therapy is showing promise for reducing inflammation, spurring recovery, and even potentially slowing aging, the principle underlying it is an old one. Since we've had ice, we've had "cryotherapy." You might have seen videos of giggling Siberian children dumping buckets of cold water over their heads while in the snow, or the Norwegian Telemark Battalion looking smug during a Cold Response exercise with U.S. Marines Black Sea Rotational Force in March 2018. The most poorly explained component of cold therapy is the goal: that you don't endeavor to muscle through the challenge. You stay calm through it and control your heart rate and the experience. And your breathing is the key.

---

4   Personal correspondence, March 11, 2018.

ARE YOU RECOVERED ENOUGH? LET'S CHECK.

Promising advancements have been made in the realm of wearable technology. Heart rate monitors and activity trackers are becoming incredibly sophisticated, and both athletes and coaches alike are making decisions based on the data these devices produce. For example, the U.S. Women's National Soccer Team wear GPS-enabled activity trackers during every game and practice, which are capable of determining whether or not an athlete is fatigued or favoring one side of her body over another. Coach Dawn Scott has made lineup changes in order to supply players more rest when the system has shown a need. "To me, recovery is such a massive aspect of overall fitness. It's what prepares you for the next session or game. If you don't recover, you start the next session tired and that sets you up for poor performance or injury," Scott told *The New York Times* on August 19, 2015.

> NBA teams sparked controversy by having starters sit out entire regular-season games in order to keep them fresh, but then the league, according to NBA.com on September 28, 2017, threatened to fine them.

For you, the change may look more like giving yourself an extra day of rest after your WHOOP strap or Oura ring overcooked it during your last WOD (workout of the day). In fact, more people than ever are relying on gadgets to tell them about the state of their bodies. For example, Paul Lamkin reported in *Forbes* that the wearable tech industry is on pace to be worth $34 billion by 2020.[5] The technologies seemingly seek to address every health question imaginable: Did I sleep enough last night? How is my posture? Is my heart rate variability what it should be? What brain waves am I emitting when I meditate?

---

5   https://www.forbes.com/sites/paullamkin/2016/02/17/wearable-tech-market-to-be-worth-34-billion-by-2020/#dd69ace3cb55.

DETOX

The findings about lactate clearance are especially relevant to breathing exercises.[6] The Horizontal Breathing and the muscle exercises you do also help you detoxify and oxygenate simultaneously. Big wave surfing pioneer and fitness guru Laird Hamilton is a big believer in detoxing and healing you can get from nature. He says that "the compression that the water creates and the movement of breathing within the body create the easiest and best detox and recovery you can get."[7]

DO THIS NOW

LEGS UP

Trainer Joe DeFranco recommends doing the Box Breathing made popular by Navy SEAL Mark Divine, author of *Unbeatable Mind* and *The Way of the SEAL*: inhale to 4 counts, hold to 4 counts, exhale to 4 counts, hold to 4 counts (or you can use 5), with legs up at a 90/90 position where hips and knees are both bent at right angles, at the end of every workout. "It makes a world of difference, and it makes a world of difference rather quickly. I can do this for five minutes and feel like a different person when I'm done," DeFranco relates. Our recommendation to add to DeFranco's prescription? Make sure you are

---

Detox with your God-given detox mechanism! Add more science. Rather than flog yourself with an intensive detox, why not just make sure the built-in one you already have is maximized. Every time you breathe diaphragmatically your liver gets a massage and the drainage system that was beautifully designed to function naturally with each breath deep cleans all your organs and lymph nodes. The best biohack you'll learn this year.

HEART RATE AND HRV

Nearly 60 studies encompassing more than 2,000 people have shown that meditative breathing techniques improve heart rate variability. Extensive data from the HeartMath Institute shows that slow, self-regulated breathing can shift the body out of a stressed emotional state and into a more regular heart rhythm.[8] This decrease in stress can be very beneficial to the recovery process and, as you'll see below in our section on resilience, an HRV may be a key determinant of whether or not you can keep your cool under fire.

---

6   Alison McConnell, author of *Respiratory Muscle Training: Theory and Practice*, recommends incorporating breathing muscles in an active recovery, since it will enable more efficient clearance of lactate and other waste from those tissues.

7   Personal correspondence, May 2019.

8   HeartMath.com, August 25, 2018.

really breathing diaphragmatically (your B-IQ score). Rx: shoulders and upper body are "soft" and relaxed. Measure your Abdominothoracic Respiratory Flexibility, and when you lie down, make sure that "position" of the breath stays the same (lower chest and belly).

MEDITATION AND RECOVERY

There are a number of reasons why meditation should be part of your active recovery. Workouts put your body into a sympathetic, unregulated state. The meditation you'll do as part of your active recovery puts you in a parasympathetic state of rest-and-digest, bringing down your heart rate, turning off your hormonal alert signals and swapping them for chemicals that instill a state of calm, and allowing your body's recovery process to begin. Results:

4. *You'll be in a better mood.* Studies published by J. D. Rooks et al. in the *Journal of Cognitive Enhancement* in 2017 recorded that athletes who performed mindfulness meditation for as little as twelve minutes a day were shown to feel better and maintain focus longer than those who simply relaxed.

5. *You'll react faster.* A study examined two groups of older adults, one that did simple stretching and strengthening exercises, and a second that did essentially the same thing but with breathing exercises added in. Within eight weeks, the group that did stretching and breathing was showing faster reaction times in cognitive tasks and performing better on memory tests, reported Neha Gothe in the *Journal of Gerontology.*[9]

6. *You'll think more clearly.* Being in an intense sympathetic go-state means your body is going to eventually cut back on your sensing things clearly. "Having the ability to hear transmissions in a dynamic environment is critical for first responders," says NYFD firefighter Jimmy Lopez, "and it's the

> Active meditation can have an interesting psychological component. Watch your reaction as you start to tire. Note your reaction as you start to tingle. Are you being close-minded? Guarded? Critical? The way you handle new situations will show up now and can give you important feedback on how you move in the world.

---

9   https://academic.oup.com/biomedgerontology/article/69/9/1109/575382/.

one thing we see decrease as the operational stress escalates." Staying alert but calm at a fire means you keep your ability to process information and make better decisions while operating in a constantly evolving environment.

7. *Meditation and creative thought?* Research from Erasmus University in Rotterdam details that just ten to twelve minutes of meditation can lead to more creative thinking. In the study, they divided up 120 people into three groups: one that followed a guided meditation, one that did a faux meditation exercise where they let their minds wander, and one that was a control. All three groups then brainstormed as many business ideas for drones as they could come up with. The three groups came up with roughly the same number of total ideas, but the meditators came up with more creative ideas across a wider variety of uses. "Better ideas, better decision making, and a better mood—all in the time it takes to drink a cup of coffee? Our study suggests that it's all true," the research team wrote when reporting their findings in 2017 in the *Harvard Business Review*.[10]

Constant revving of your engine, without the waxing and waning of stress that allows you to "cool off," is what is causing intense problems with modern stress. An acute spike of stress, then a return to calm is actually better than an ongoing stressed state which is a chronic sympathetic state. Cal Dietz, founder of RPR, explains: "Because our life stressors are a constant bombardment in our daily lives, the body is unaware of when the stressful stimuli will subside. This makes it impossible to return to normal and causes the neuromusculoskeletal system to look at long-term solutions to survive. There is an increase in resting heart rate, labored (chest) breathing, and the development of compensations."[11]

A MINDFUL ADVANTAGE: 12 MINUTES OF MEDITATION MAKES A BIG DIFFERENCE FOR DIVISION I FOOTBALL PLAYERS

A breath-focused meditation can improve your mood and your focus, even in the midst of physical and mental stress. That's the key takeaway from a 2017 study conducted by J. D. Rooks and his colleagues at the University of Miami. In it, the school's psychology department spent four weeks working with one hundred foot-

---

10   https://hbr.org/.

11   https://www.elitefts.com/education/rpr-wake-up-your-true-performance-potential/.

ball players at "The U" during four weeks of preseason training. It was a tough time, with two-a-day practices taking a toll on their bodies and worries over winning a starting position stressing their minds. Researchers split the players into two groups, with half learning relaxation techniques and the other half engaging in a mindfulness meditation that required them to pay close attention to their breathing and to the present moment. The interventions were short. Athletes practiced the techniques for just twelve minutes a day. By the end, athletes in both the relaxation and meditation groups showed improvements. They were less stressed and in better moods. But there was a clear winner. "Those in the meditation group, if they had practiced often, showed considerable mental resilience, with higher scores than the other athletes in either group on the measures of both attention and mood," reported Gretchen Reynolds in a write-up of the study that appeared in *The New York Times*.[12] Bottom line: meditation with attention to breathing outpaces simple relaxation techniques when it comes to an effective cooldown, but either is better than the "nothing" that most people do to wind down their workouts.

Becoming aware of your breath is the most fundamental of all awareness practices. It's literally step one. With that control, you can practice other qualities you want to exhibit: maintaining good humor amid challenges, staying in the fight when things get tough. With time, those practices become who you are. "We are what we repeatedly do," goes a quote often misattributed to Aristotle. (It was actually written by Will Durant in an examination of Aristotle's work.)

IN BLUE, OUT RED

During Game 7 of the 2012 Eastern Conference Finals between the Miami Heat and Boston Celtics, cameras caught a glimpse into the mind and breath of a champion. Viewers could see LeBron James taking slow breaths as he sat on the team's bench during a time-out.

Meditation and breathwork have expanded into other professional leagues. "I love to meditate in the morning," says former

---

12   June 21, 2017.

Chicago Cubs manager Joe Maddon. "To me, it's very, very helpful to just really get my mind right for the course of the day. So that when you do come to the moments, you have to make a decision that you feel convicted in that decision, and that is based on what you do prior to, during and then after."[13]

Maddon's Cubs made headlines in 2016 for wearing shirts that read "In blue, out red"—a reminder from team mental performance coach Darnell McDonald to relax during inhales and let go of stress on exhales.[14] Coaches like McDonald used to be a novelty in the league; but as of the 2018 season, 27 of 30 MLB teams had a mental performance coach on their rosters. The macho world of football has been a little slower in coming around to the power of breathwork and meditation, but received a kick in the pants when the Seattle Seahawks used yoga and meditation to power their way to a Super Bowl win in 2013.[15] Today the San Francisco 49ers, Indianapolis Colts, and Atlanta Falcons are also using mindfulness techniques in their training.[16] Plenty of individual sport athletes have used attentive breathing and meditation practices to powerful effect. Dr. Jeff Leiter has added breathing exercises to his protocol for hockey players, stressing that, "Hockey requires you to have high bursts of high energy, then being seated, usually tipped forward, leaning on your knees. You are trying not to mull about your last shot while being prepped to shoot out of the gate at any second."[17]

IS MEDITATION THE KEY TO SEEING THAT CURVEBALL?

You've heard that meditation can help you see things more clearly. Well, a research team led by Katherine MacLean at the University of California, Davis, sought to put the idea to the test. They recruited sixty participants who were aged between twenty and seventy-one, and who had to be ready to make a commitment:

13   Quoted by Matthew Peaslee in *The Herald Star,* November 3, 2016.

14   *USA Today,* February 21, 2016.

15   *ESPN The Magazine,* August 21, 2013.

16   *The Ringer,* August 15, 2017.

17   Personal correspondence, May 12, 2018.

all were required to abstain from tobacco and recreational drugs for three months leading up to the study, and then continue to stay away from drugs or alcohol for the study's three-month duration. During those three months, participants lived in a mountain retreat northwest of Fort Collins, Colorado, where they received instructions and practiced meditating or solitude for up to five hours a day. Following the study, tests indicated that the meditators were actually seeing the world more clearly. "Reliable improvements in visual discrimination" is how the study authors put it, adding that their data "suggests that mental training of attention on non-visual perceptions (e.g., sensations of breathing and mental events) generalizes to improved visual perception of task-relevant stimuli." Your takeaway: by observing your breath, then, you'll become better at observing the world around you too.

INCREASE THAT GRAY MATTER THROUGH MEDITATION!

Harvard Neuroscientist Sara Lazar discovered something curious. In a study of long-term meditators, she saw that fifty-year-old meditators had as much gray matter in their prefrontal cortex (a region of the brain associated with decision-making and memory) as a typical twenty-five-year-old. That's a big deal, because gray matter tends to decline as people age. But there was the chance that the fifty-year-olds just had more gray matter to begin with. So she ran a second study. This time she recruited a group of thirty-five people and split them into two groups. One was a control group, the other underwent eight weeks of mindfulness-based stress reduction training which included breath awareness training. After the eight weeks, Lazar's team noticed clear differences: the brains of those who'd been meditating had thickened in four important areas, including regions responsible for learning, memory, cognition, and emotional regulation. Interestingly, their amygdala region shrank, and meditators reported feeling less stressed overall. The results would indicate that meditation and breath awareness build the mind just as physical training builds the body. "Mindfulness is just like exercise. It's a form of mental exercise, really," Lazar told *The Washington Post*.[18]

18   May 26, 2015. https://hms.harvard.edu/news/harvard-neuroscientist.

> *Being able to up- and downregulate at will—to make sure that your central nervous system is ready to go—is the most important, but most underestimated factor in training today. It is, really, the magic pill.*

MEDITATION FOR INNER GAME

Meditation can help you mentally detox in that you will let go of the stress that your body was holding and of which you weren't conscious. You may shake or tingle, you may laugh, or shed a tear. All these should be without judgment. It is simply your body shaking off stress in the same way, as we already pointed out, animals do in the wild.

You may find that you are able to access a place that feels spiritual. It is an intensely comforting moment, when you feel "flow" or sense you can "hear" your intuition. This is a feeling you will practice accessing. It feels divine—even magical—but it is something you will learn to access with practice. During this time just "watch" and try not to overthink things.

I have called this practice "meditation for people who can't meditate." Why? Well, after the breathing exercises you will find that it's easier for your brain to follow your body and calm down. Definitely more effective than trying to get your body to be still because your brain tells it to do so. Will this help you go deeper or be able to do other types of meditation? Absolutely.

Finally, while you don't have to do anything specific to get these benefits, the movement of your body when breathing hard and using your diaphragm detoxifies your body.[19] There is nothing magical about it. The diaphragm's movement rids your body of waste products like lymph faster than any diet or detox rituals. It's mind-numbingly simple. Most people ignore the fact that the fastest built-in detox system is the body itself. And don't forget to drink plenty of water afterward.

-meditation-not-only-reduces-stress-heres-how-changes-your-brain

19   Although if you have access to a salt cave or halotherapy salt room like Salthaus in New York City (https://www.salthausny.com) you can multitask your meditation with dry salty air that has been shown to absorb bacteria and pollutants.

WHAT ARE THE RESULTS?

Endurance and breathing research show that working out the breathing muscles apart from your sport is what takes them to the level of exhaustion (overload) and makes them stronger. The fatigue you'll experience is exactly the same, though you won't have the same burning or heavy feeling you are used to when working on "exterior muscles." Having your body (hips) move with the breath in an exaggerated way helps you relearn how movement and breathing go hand in hand, and it keeps your pace even when you get tired.

This push when you are tired is part of training yourself to keep going when you are fatigued. The translation into your sport not only will be that you have practiced recovering but you'll be more tenacious (have more heart) in moments when you have to dig deep.

> *Practicing and repeating the stress of pushing your breathing muscles has complex results. Simply put, breathing hard while competing will not seem as uncomfortable. It will not interfere as much with your experiencing the situation as stressful.*

EXERCISES

PART ONE

1. Keep breathing through your mouth for this entire first part. Lying on your back, with nothing bulky under your head, put one hand on your belly button and the other on the top of your chest, by your collarbones. Breathe through your mouth for this part of the exercise. Inhale and expand your belly. At this time, the breath can be just a simple belly breath or you might be starting to feel your lower ribs and sides move as well. When you are "full," take a second inhale and push your shoulders back against the floor, feeling as if you were opening up the top of your chest by your collarbones, then add a "sip" of air there (this feeling should be as

if you filled a container, then added a bit more to fill it to the very top). Make sure that your hips are moving: on the belly inhale you are creating space at your lower back, which you will decrease on the exhale (your lower back flattens against the floor).

2. Find a rhythm that suits you, and stick to it. You should be able to find or "drop down" into this rhythm with more ease each time.

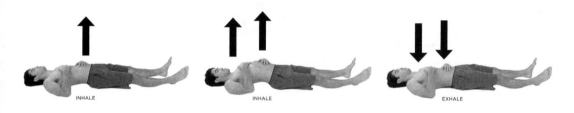

3. No matter what happens, just encourage yourself calmly and firmly to continue breathing. Any peculiar or uncomfortable sensations will lessen each time you practice, and the benefits are priceless. Understand that you may hit a wall. Some people hit it after twenty breaths, others significantly later.[20] In fact, the first few times you practice this active meditation you will hit the same kind of wall that you do when you work out. You will hear yourself make excuses about why you want to stop. Keep going. If you feel a little tingling, that's OK! Just encourage yourself to keep going, and remind yourself you are doing well and are almost done. Believe that there will be a moment when you get to the "other side."

TROUBLESHOOT

Be careful that the upper breath does not become bigger than the lower one. People sometimes relapse to an upper breath style because it is "easier"; the challenge is to stay low.

---

20 Want something to aspire to? UFC Champ Jake Ellenberger has practiced this intense two-part breath for half an hour.

PART TWO

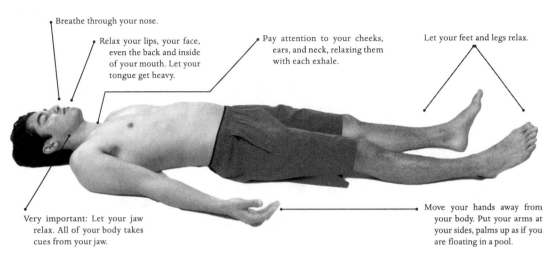

Breathe through your nose.

Relax your lips, your face, even the back and inside of your mouth. Let your tongue get heavy.

Pay attention to your cheeks, ears, and neck, relaxing them with each exhale.

Let your feet and legs relax.

Very important: Let your jaw relax. All of your body takes cues from your jaw.

Move your hands away from your body. Put your arms at your sides, palms up as if you are floating in a pool.

Now you are going to switch to a big, gentle inhale and a big, gentle exhale. With each inhale, let yourself float a little higher, and with each exhale, let yourself sink a little deeper. Continue doing mental body scans from time to time to make sure you are not holding tension anywhere. You may be surprised to discover that you may have a place that is always tensed, so much so that you have become accustomed to it. Try to move your mind away from thinking; simply keep your attention on your physical sensations. By "keep your attention on" we mean observe your body breathe as if you were watching another person, noting sensations but trying not to figure them out.

KEEP IN MIND

- Make sure you are *not* narrowing your middle when you take the top breath. Keep your belly wide and "add" to it.
- Make sure that the timing of the inhale and exhale stay the same. Two counts for the inhale, two counts for the exhale.
- This is not hyperventilation; while you are breathing hard, you are in control of both the inhale and the exhale.

Drop all language. Most of us spend too much time in our heads and eyes (looking and working "forward")—meaning we are constantly taking in visual information and breathing with our shoulders. "Moving your breathing down" means you "turn off" your brain. While you are in this calming (possibly trance-like) part of the meditation, "drop" all language—notice thoughts or feelings but try not to put words or meaning to them. This takes practice.

- The sound of your breathing should help you keep the cadence the same. All you need to do is find a rhythm you can fall into.
- Keep breathing in and out through your nose during the dynamic first part. The sound of your breath and feeling of quantity of air going in and out of your body is important.
- There should be two distinct inhales, and the second one is small. It is not one long breath. Your shoulders just push back against the floor slightly.

FREQUENTLY ASKED QUESTIONS

Q: If my back is moving away from the floor on the inhale, doesn't that make for a smaller "big" breath?

A: *The movement of your hips and your lower back coming away from the floor helps with the rhythm of the breathing by changing the cue of the shoulder movement to a middle body expansion. The movement of your entire body makes this exercise feel like a whole-body one that has a therapeutic "shaking" component to it. (You may want to check out Bradford Keeney's book, Shaking Medicine.) The movement also allows your psoas to be part of the process. A true measure of whether you are taking a big breath comes from the B-IQ.*

WHY DOES BREATHWORK FEEL SO GOOD?

Many people spend time bracing themselves, often just grinding their teeth trying not to emote or get visibly irritated. If you check yourself, you may discover that you do this even in small ways, and more often than you realize. As we pointed out earlier, animals get to shake it off, or growl and not take it personally. For us, the discomfort accumulates and we distort, deny, and self-medicate.

Strangely enough, we can schedule in our "shaking it off." If you have enough irritability, anger, or sadness accumulated, it might come out like a "release." So, what does a release feel like? It can feel like a deeply satisfying sigh or even an all-out, several-minutes-long cry and wail you've been stifling for years. It can be a giggle that comes out of nowhere. Whatever it is, don't dampen it down or stop it—that's the exact opposite of what you want to do. Why does this happen? Some people call this an "activation" or a "cathartic release." Some reasons for why this happens are:

1. In a prone position you can take a Belly/Horizontal Parasympathetic Breath even if you never take one standing up. It's the one position when most people breathe in an anatomically congruous way (usually because they are not sucking in their belly or bracing).

2. You are probably looking up at a blank ceiling, so it's easier to turn your attention inward rather than be processing visual information. (In fact, in classic psychoanalytic therapy this prone position puts you in a less inhibited neutral state so you can see what comes to mind.)

3. Your exhale is better because of gravity in a prone position; therefore, your inhale can be better.

4. You are unbracing. You don't need your breathing muscles for posture; you should use them for breathing.

5. You have permission to do nothing (without being called lazy)—meaning you can actually pause and allow yourself to be in the present.

6. You can't multitask. Yes, that means your phone should be put away.

7. You can belly breathe without shame. Regardless of your body type, how ripped you are or aren't, it's easier to let your guard down in a prone position and not feel like you have to flex or suck it in.

8. If breathing is enthusiastic, you get a boost of endorphins, and your stress hormone cortisol goes down.

> "Breathwork is life changing—whether reducing stress, controlling or eliminating disease symptoms, improving sleep, or even being a better person at work and at home. I truly believe that the breath is the key to unlocking our bodies' abilities to heal themselves and perform at optimal capacity. By changing our physiology and being fully accessible to anyone, breathwork has the potential for wide-ranging benefits."
>
> — Dr. Tanya Bentley, Cofounder, CEO, Health & Human Performance Foundation

9. Massage of belly breath feels good, especially to the digestive system where the second biggest serotonin receptor sites are located.

10. You are doing a detox by using breathing muscles in the middle of your body more. You are flushing lymph and waste products out of your body.

WRITE IT DOWN

Green Beret Lt. Col. Scott Mann[21] is Danny Patton in *Last Out*; he turned his compelling story into a play in which he must transition quickly from moments of rage to those of tenderness. Scott's nonprofit, The Heroes Journey, funded by Scott and his wife, Monty Mann, is dedicated to helping our military men and women find their voice and tell their story in transition with free books, workshops, and virtual training.

Journaling before and after these exercises is very important so that you remember your feelings and the wisps of thought that arose. If you feel strong emotions or thoughts or anxiety bubble up, don't dig in your heels. Your reaction to things getting tough is to hold on tighter, to keep control. This truly is a mind/body exercise because while you want to fall into a rhythm and push yourself, you have to learn to let go at the same time. Bringing awareness to these thoughts and feelings gives them meaning; make a mental note but don't judge or try to control. Sometimes as you get closer to an uncomfortable feeling or thought, you'll experience an upsurge of anxiety. Rather than back away from it, lean into it. See if you can tap into it. This will make more sense as you do the meditation.

> *Even a short ten-minute active recovery breathing meditation can bring your blood pressure down and change your mood. Adding a breathing active meditation should be your first priority after a hard day, regardless of what that day entailed.*

---

21   http://www.theheroesjourney.org.

HOW TO USE BREATHING MEDITATION
THERAPEUTICALLY AS AN EXERCISE FOR YOUR MIND

1. Keep a notepad next to you. Write down what comes up, and don't judge; just bring awareness to the fact that this particular thought or memory is meaningful in some way. At some point you'll be able to "connect the dots," but for now, just accept them. They don't have to make sense right away. If you forget one, don't worry; if it's important, it will come up again.

2. When you are doing the relaxing second part of the breath, don't search for answers or try to overthink. Just let yourself feel "open," as if you were taking suggestions. Dropping all language is harder than you'd imagine. The brain is constantly trying to compartmentalize and log experiences. "Staying in sensation" is something to practice that is a brain and meditation exercise.

3. Switch it up by setting an intention, which means you have a goal in mind. Let "it"—getting through a hard time, putting the past behind you—whatever "it" is, go. Listen to the "but" or "what if" type thoughts that enter your mind. Bring awareness to them (shine daylight on them), then see how you can dismantle them, practically, in your everyday life.

4. Listen to your intuition. Does something someone said to you ring true; do you have a memory surface, one you'd forgotten about?

5. Get perspective. Get out of your own head. Talk to yourself about the bigger picture.

6. End by repeating something inspiring. "This too will pass," or "Let go, let God," or anything that inspires patience and being gentle with yourself.

7. Use the breathing meditation as a tool. Use the stress of a hard workout or a trying day to train yourself to face challenging situations.

17

BETWEEN YOUR EARS: BREATHING TECHNIQUES TO MASTER YOUR INNER GAME

WHAT'S BETWEEN YOUR EARS?

What's between your ears? Everything that has to do with your mental health, how you react to stress, arousal control, and your inner game. How resilient are you? How do you respond to injury? Finally, what skills do you need to transition from field to stage? We'll cover all that in the next pages.

MENTAL HEALTH

Michael Phelps, the most decorated Olympian of all time and now a mental health advocate, told *Everyday Health,* "There are times when I struggle with identity because for so many people, all they see me as is a swimmer. Honestly, that's when a lion's breath does come into play."

OK, let's be clear about this. Breathing exercises alone cannot heal the suicidal depression that American swimmer Michael Phelps admitted to after two counts of DUI, but it can be the pause that allows a person to reflect and formulate a plan of self-care.[1]

EVERY BREATHING STATE HAS AN EMOTIONAL STATE (AND VICE VERSA)

Researchers have repeatedly observed that certain breathing patterns correspond with certain emotional states. For example,

---

1   Robinson, Katie. "Michael Phelps's Favorite De-stress Technique Is So Simple, Anyone Can Do It," *Everyday Health*, March 2019.

there is a positive correlation between anxiety and breathing frequency, meaning that people who feel more anxious tend to breathe more rapidly and from the upper chest.[2]

The amount of research showing that breathing can influence mental state is too compelling to omit, although it deserves much more space. The bi-directionality of the breath means that it affects one's mental state and, consequently, mental state affects our breathing. Belisa's journey from psychologist to breathing teacher came from understanding how what previous renowned researchers were studying related to psychiatric disorders and breathing patterns.[3] She took her specialization in IQ testing and child psychology and filled in the gap by adding instructions to help with change. Which leads us to being right here, right now, with you.

THE BIOMECHANICS OF STRESS

A relationship between emotional well-being and the quality of one's breathing mechanics has always been evident, but complex. Part of the problem in understanding it is the strict division between pulmonary health and how the quality and location of breath affects the nervous system. Another issue is how, in talking about the mechanism of breathing and breathing science in relation to emotions, the conversation often becomes almost mystical.

What's indisputably true is this: Stressed out, depressed, and anxious people often have bad breathing mechanics and patterns. And people with bad breathing mechanics are often stressed out, depressed, and anxious. The question then becomes: Which came first, the stressor or the stress-inducing breathing pattern? The answer is extremely difficult to parse and—honestly—doesn't always matter. However, what does matter is this: if you break that pattern

---

2   Homma, Ikuo and Masaoka, Yuri. "Breathing rhythms and emotions." *Experimental Physiology.*

3   E.g., Robert Fried, author of *The Psychology and Physiology of Breathing: In Behavioral Medicine Clinical Psychology and Psychiatry*, studied with one of my favorites, the world-renowned psychotherapist Albert Ellis (Rational Emotive Behavioral Therapy), who is known for being confrontational, headstrong, and steadfastly rational.

of shallow, erratic Vertical Breathing, a cascade of benefits often results, including a significant decrease in stress and anxiety.

Nevertheless, it is both ironic and astounding that athletes (competitive or tactical), often heralded for their physical and mental toughness, may be more vulnerable to these emotional disorders than the general population. Many athletes have stepped forward to talk about their mental health problems; e.g., MLB All-Star Alex Rodriguez, Dwayne "The Rock" Johnson, Serena Williams, four-time Super Bowl champion Terry Bradshaw, MMA champions Georges St.-Pierre and Ronda Rousey, boxer Oscar De La Hoya, NFL All-Pros Brandon Marshall, Alonzo Spellman, and Ricky Williams, Olympic gold medalist swimmer Amanda Beard, Olympic diver Wendy Williams, former Detroit Piston Brian Williams, Olympic gold medalist swimmer Ian Crocker, former Minnesota Timberwolves guard Kendall Gill, and Olympic gold medalist diver Greg Louganis.

NFL quarterback and sportscaster Terry Bradshaw, whom I interviewed in 2016 for a magazine article, confided:
"I would just run. When I felt bad, all I knew was that I should put my sneakers on and move. It was instinct. The endorphins from the run made me feel better...I didn't realize that the problem was much more than a couple miles of running could fix."

While the physiological makeup of athletes does not make them any more prone to mental health problems than their nonathletic counterparts, their *circumstances* do; e.g. loss of identity after injuries ended a stellar athletic career. More than half of the players who committed suicide were between their late twenties and late forties, and 15 percent did so within two years after their major league careers had ended.[4] Disordered breathing can cause more preperformance anxiety in athletes; in fact, fear of breathlessness is paramount. Often performance stress is the entry point to start the conversation.

The Mindbody Prescription by John Sarno (made popular by his patient and radio shock-jock Howard Stern) speaks to the integration of breathing and therapy when dealing with emotional and physical pain. Several experienced breathworkers, including psychiatrist Stan Grof and psychologist Jim Morningstar, have been pas-

---

4   In a landmark study in 1987, Loren Coleman, a researcher at the Human Services Development Institute at the University of Southern Maine and the author of *Suicide Clusters*, found that seventy-seven Major League Baseball players had taken their lives since the early part of the century.

sionate in their teaching how breathing helps heal trauma (from natural disasters to war).[5]

Studies and articles nowadays pop up quite frequently that look at how breathing practice and meditation can help alleviate symptoms of depression and anxiety (and let's be clear on this also: this in no way means that I propose that clinical depression or anxiety should be treated with breathing or meditation exclusively). Places such as The Huberman Lab (www.hubermanlab.com) in San Francisco are making great strides in research regarding mechanisms and biology of fear. Traumatic brain injury and combat/transitional stress are a hot topic of discussion.

One explanation of states like anxiety, depression, and PTSD is that they are all forms of being "stuck." Essentially, a person can get trapped in a state of being over- or under-activated—or vacillate between the two. As a result, they're not able to respond normally to life as it happens. Research indicates that two neurotransmitters can wield influence over this activation level in our minds: gamma-aminobutyric acid (GABA) and glutamate. The two act in opposition to each another. Glutamate is an excitatory compound, while GABA is inhibitory. The levels of these two chemicals are modulated by your autonomic nervous system, a lizard brain–like network of nerves throughout the body communicating with the brain. The network includes the vagus nerves, two matching nerves that wrap down from the brain into each side of your body. Depressed people typically have low GABA. But if the vagus nerve is stimulated, it will release GABA. And recent research shows that activities like controlled breathing or yoga can stimulate the vagus nerve, and cause a cascade of other effects as a result. Randomized controlled trial

> ### IS HBOT THE SOLUTION?
>
> Hyperbaric oxygen therapy is one of the most powerful ways to decrease inflammation, according to Dr. Scott Sherr, Director of Integrative Hyperbaric Medicine and Health Optimization at Hyperbaric Medical Solutions. Dr. Scherr has found that HBOT decreases inflammation, accelerates wound healing, and optimizes both physical and mental performance.

---

5   One of the newest treatments for trauma is ART—Accelerated Resolution Therapy. Lead ART trainer, Dr. Diego Hernandez of Tampa, Florida, has found ART to be particularly helpful with resolving PTSD symptoms with veterans, palliative care patients, and motorcycle accident victims.

studies[6] have found that people suffering from anxiety, depression, or addiction who performed breathing activities or yoga for twelve weeks saw GABA levels in their brains normalize. They also experienced a corresponding decrease in depressive symptoms, and scored better on examinations of their tranquility, vitality, and physical energy.[7]

DO THIS NOW

Lion's Breath. To do it, you take in a big, full abdominothoracic breath, and then exhale forcefully, making a *haaaa* sound (or even a roar if you want to really get in the mood) in the back of your throat. The reason you may experience immediate relief is the stretch it gives your tongue and neck, which, given the amount of talking and unnatural craning we do in our modern posture, releases tension.

INNER GAME

"When you want to succeed as much as you want to breathe, then you will be successful," said Eric Thomas, "the hip hop preacher," minister, author, and speaker.[8] Belisa often references him, then rephrases, "When you want to BREATHE as much as you want to succeed, then you will be successful." The truth is it is hard to have anyone talk about inner game without mentioning breathing, but now you have *the how.* So, let's talk about inner game.

First of all, how do you define inner game for yourself? Staying balanced and focused despite the "noise" around you? Staying optimistic regardless of your last play? While these are classic thoughts in the arena of sports, they are metaphors of life as well.

---

6   Basically, the gold standard of research methodologies.

7   Streeter, et al. "Effects of Yoga on Thalamic Gamma-Aminobutyric Acid, Mood and Depression: Analysis of Two Randomized Controlled Trials." *Neuropsychiatry.* http://www.jneuropsychiatry.org/peer-review/effects-of-yoga -on-thalamic-gammaaminobutyric-acid-mood-and-depression-analysis-of-two -randomized-controlled-trials-12856.html.

8   You might want to check out his album *Dr. Thomas* for more inspiration.

The Shut Up and *The Listen* response	*The Next Play Mentality* approach	*The Injury-Proofing* attitude

WHAT EXACTLY IS INNER GAME?

1. ***The Shut Up*** and ***The Listen*** response: "In training, you listen to your body. In competition, you tell your body to shut up," says four-time CrossFit Games champion Rich Froning,[9] author of *First: What It Takes to Win.* Working on your inner game means you pay attention to developing both: when your body is teetering toward injury and you need to pull back, and when you are slacking and need to dig deeper.

2. ***The Next Play Mentality*** approach: Your ability to bounce back from one bad play or loss and move on without self-defeating negative self-talk that bleeds into your next shot. Coined by Coach Mike Krzyzewski, he describes this approach in his engaging YouTube video, "The Concept of 'Next Play,'" in which he recounts when he came to "the realization that, no matter what just happened, I've got to be really good at the next thing."

3. ***The Injury-Proofing*** attitude: Being able to come back from an injury and play with all the confidence you had before you got hurt. In *MIZZOU*, the magazine of the University of Missouri Alumni Association, Dr. Aaron Gray, a physician for the university's athletes, says that fear of being hurt again can actually prevent

> "Sometimes when I make my routines I get in a very special stage of meditation, and this is beautiful because I am able to exercise and I'm able to totally clean my mind and keep myself in the present moment. When you control your breath you can actually control yourself mentally and physically; you can really understand your fears and your emotional stress."—Rickson Gracie, holder of a ninth-degree red belt, the highest rank awarded to any currently living practitioner of Brazilian jiu-jitsu, as quoted by Tony Pacenski (author of *A Story of Invisible Power*).

---

9 https://www.boxrox.com/rich-fronings-most-inspiring-quotes/

athletes from recovering completely. Good inner game is the opposite of that. Perhaps elite obstacle course racer Amelia Boone summed it up best when she said of her return to racing after suffering a broken femur: "I am not going to run away from fear. Instead I am running toward it."[10]

Inner game, then, is all of these and much more. It's being self-confident, effortlessly focusing on the task at hand without dwelling on what happened before or what will happen later. It's not allowing past injuries to create limiting assumptions; it's disallowing self-defeating chatter in your head; it's refusing to be plagued by self-doubts when the going gets rough. Your inner game is something you should be working on continually.

MANAGING AROUSAL:
WHAT IS AN "ADRENALINE DUMP"
(AND HOW CAN I BEAT IT?)

There's no official medical diagnosis for an adrenaline dump (which doctors prefer to call an "adrenaline rush"), but the experience is something that the tactical community and MMA fighters know all too well. You're in a fight and you're amped to eleven. Your hearing is often the first thing to go (a sensation called auditory exclusion). For some, this means they hear nothing—not even the gunshots produced by their own weapon. For others, they'll hear the wrong thing. All of this is why a number of fire departments are teaching techniques designed to keep

> "A real-life tactical situation has risk and adrenaline and resilience that can't be factored in the way you can in combat sports. You have to reverse engineer breathing and fear because if you even consider you are the zebra, you are fucked. There is the psychology of fear and the biology of fear; breathing as it relates to both is a massive epiphany. We need to practice it."[11]
>
> — Tony Blauer, Founder, Blauer Tactical Systems

10   Quoted by Lara McGlashan in her March 6, 2019 article on MuscleandPerformance.com about the legendary runner who is considered the world's best Tough Mudder Champion.

11   Interview, April 28, 2019.

firefighters calm under pressure so that they don't hear the wrong orders. One can also lose peripheral vision, which is a big problem in a situation where danger can come at you from any direction. Young MMA fighters often respond to adrenaline dumps by going all out at the start of a fight—and running out of gas quickly. Deep breathing is the antidote to all of this. By bringing your attention to your breath, you'll get clarity and choices rather than panic and stress hormones.

HOW A HIGHER HRV KEEPS YOU CALM UNDER FIRE

Lea Hildebrandt and her team of researchers at the Max Planck Institute for Human Cognitive and Brain Sciences in Leipzig, Germany, sought to examine the relationship between Heart Rate Variability and how people react when they feel they are under threat. After taking baseline HRV measurements of more than three hundred people, scientists used VR devices to put the subjects into a creepy-as-hell virtual world known as Room 101. The room looks like something out of a Queens of the Stone Age video: it's dark, gray, and infested with spiders.[12] But participants don't know that at the start. Their experience begins in a seemingly harmless (if poorly lit) environment filled with crates, where they are instructed to search and find little canisters strewn about. But things quickly get weird. Gunshots go off. Crates explode and there are lots of spiders. In the grand finale, the floor collapses. With each threat, wearable sensors placed on the skin measure the person's arousal level. The result? Both people with high and low HRVs reacted to the onset of threats such as a gunshot or an alarm; however, those with high HRVs quickly returned to their baseline level. They had recog-

> I was invited to teach Breathing for Warriors by Rickson black belt Henry "The Professor" Atkins at Dynamix MMA in Los Angeles. Smack in the front, with the flexibility of a ten-year-old gymnast and thick salt-and-pepper hair slicked back, was a large man with the focus of a hawk. For the entire three-hour workshop, he hardly blinked; comedian Joey "Coco" Diaz has a heart of gold and a sense of humor that would make the Queen's guard blush and he is a blue belt in jiu-jitsu. Both Henry and Joey are staunch advocates of the mechanics of breathing.

12   Want to "experience" Room 101 yourself? Go to: https://youtu.be /Lnl8opbaP4U.

nized the threat, then calmed down and moved on. Those with low HRV stayed in an elevated state of alert, becoming more alarmed and jumpy. The conclusion: higher HRVs are associated with better decision-making and greater calm in times of stress or emergency. And slow, controlled breathing is a proven technique for improving HRV.

PLAYING DEAD

The freeze response is also known as "tonic immobility," which roughly translates as, "you tense up everywhere and feel as if you can't move." Scientists believe the reaction is related to the natural instinct some animals exhibit ("playing dead") when they feel they are in a fight they can't win. In humans, the freeze response doesn't get the same attention that its cousin "fight or flight" receives, which means it's also less understood. To gain more insight into it, researchers recruited about four hundred people in and around Ohio State University in Columbus, Ohio, evaluating them for more than two years through both psychological tests and blood tests that examined specific biomarkers, and published their results in the *Journal of Behavior Therapy and Experimental Psychiatry* in 2007. Participants were informed that they would be asked to breathe a mixture of CO_2-enriched air. When they were told this, they were also warned of numerous potential consequences of breathing the air, like dizziness, breathlessness, and chest pain. Before the test, almost none of the participants believed they would freeze up under stress. But once the masks were placed on and the people were asked to breathe the bad air for twenty seconds, one out of every eight reported feelings of immobility. Scientists noticed two patterns in the data: those who froze up were generally more anxious and had higher baseline levels of cortisol. Which makes now a great time to remind you that meditation is an effective way to lower cortisol levels. The rule: breathe; don't freeze.

KEEP IN MIND

Your breathing is the control for your nervous system. It can keep you calm when things are hectic around you, and vice versa, it can rile you up when things are relatively calm around you. Think about how you feel when you wake up from a dream: your heart and breath might be altered although you were just asleep under your blanket. Your nervous system doesn't distinguish between the ramping up that comes from responding to an ambush and a nightmare of one when you are asleep. Being aware of what you do when sleeping, whether it's nightmares or teeth grinding, can give you an idea of what is still unsettled in your unconscious, regardless of how together you seem to be during the day. Dredging that up, dealing with it, and continuing to better yourself is lifelong.

RESILIENCE

From Belisa: Jason Brezler, decorated Marine, Brooklyn-based firefighter, and founder of Leadership Under Fire, defined resilience succinctly for me: "Resilience is the ability to absorb both micro and macro failure for the greater good of the mission."[13]

When I first started teaching, it was not the yoga community or the "worried well" that invited me to talk. It was a population where resilience is critical: first responders (e.g., EMS, call dispatchers, drug enforcement agents, firefighters, policemen, and military personnel). Caregivers are first responders as well. It was about this time that I met Gaby Camargo, wife of Romy Camargo, Chief Warrant Officer (Ret.), U.S. Army. During his third deployment to Afghanistan in 2008, Camargo's mission had been canceled. Dedicated to service, he volunteered to do a humanitarian mission. Romy's detachment was ambushed during the mission, and he was struck in the neck by a sniper's bullet. Camargo arrived at Walter Reed National Military Medical Center on his wife Gaby's birthday. Gaby has been com-

"Having experience in lifting and martial arts gave me a better sense of a diaphragmatic breath, and it helped me go from a wheelchair to a prosthetic," says Officer Byron Branch of the Dayton Police Department. Member of the US national wheelchair team, Branch says that "BJJ is the full-body equivalent of wheelchair fencing. With fencing I focus on wearing out the opponent; it's about reading the breath and efficacy of movement."[14]

---

13   Personal communication, March 10, 2018.
14   Interview on March 30, 2019.

pared to a lioness in her ferocity and dedication to Romy's rehab. Together they created Stay in Step, a facility in Tampa, Florida, that provides some of the highest-quality and cutting-edge services for spinal cord injury in the world.

BROTHERHOOD AS A RESILIENCE TOOL

Resilience is a topic that comes up at nearly every peak performance workshop. Then we end up talking about Sebastian Junger's bestseller *Tribe*, or the number of wildfires our firefighters are dealing with as we speak, or sociopolitical issues like the number of injured vets returning Stateside. Force Blue is the brainchild of Rudy Reyes and Jim Ritterhoff, who strive to provide "mission therapy" to former combat divers—individuals in whom governments around the world have invested millions to create the best possible underwater and maritime operators—by retraining, retooling, and deploying them on missions of conservation, preservation, and restoration. "Breathing, underwater or on land, tactical or social, is the soul of every mission," says Reyes, a former Recon Marine who had struggled with PTSD and depression since returning home from multiple tours in Iraq and Afghanistan. He clarifies: "Breath underlies mechanical coordination; it is also the very essence of what connects one human being to another."[15]

> **READ THIS:**
>
> After a Japanese torpedo struck the *Indianapolis*, more than nine hundred men died, a number of them eaten by sharks. Authors Lynn Vincent and Sara Vladic (*Indianapolis: The True Story of the Worst Sea Disaster in U.S. Naval History and the Fifty-Year Fight to Exonerate an Innocent Man*) described with harrowing and riveting detail the bravery and resilience of the survivors.

TOUGH VS. RESILIENT

Know the difference between tough and resilient? "To me," said Rob Martin, Deputy Fire Chief, Kitchener, Canada, "tough is rigid and inflexible. Sure it can take a lot of abuse, likely withstand an incredible amount of stress. But it has no range of emotion. Someone who is resilient can withstand the same amount of stress but moves with it. They have the range of emotion to be empathetic

---

15   Personal correspondence, April 28, 2018.

in an emergency and still be a high performer."[16]

Brendan Cawley, an active-duty fireman at Ladder Company 27 in New York City, manages to mix humor and inspiration into his first few minutes of an account of jumping out of a fifth-story window on "Black Sunday at the FDNY MPI Performance Leader's Course on April 4, 2019."[17] Prior to his presentation, the audience hears the radio transmission as a fire goes wrong and firefighters facing 700-degree heat fall from the top windows to their deaths. Cawley seems unaffected by the awe he inspires as he describes in eerie detail the sprawl of bodies at the base of the building before his own jump. One of the first questions he asked when waking up at the hospital was how long before he could go back to work.

Right now employers, police and fire departments, and the military are looking for ways to accurately gauge resiliency. It's easy to understand why: resilient people don't give up even when the odds seem impossibly stacked against them. As J. C. Glick, former Army Ranger and combat veteran, and author of *Meditations of an Army Ranger: A Warrior Philosophy for Everyone*, points out: "It is in that moment, when you choose to adapt instead of quit, where resilience is born."[18] In a personal communication, he expanded on the subject of mental preparation, a term he learned from Mike Pannone, a former SFOD operator: "Mental preparation can be trained; it is deliberate. It is like doing PT, cleaning your weapon, or practicing an obstacle course. Unlike mindset, it is practiced so you can use it when you need it. Mental preparation silences that little voice inside your head that hurts your resiliency; it is that voice that lies when you are faced with the unknown and tells you that you can't. If you don't practice on the thinking about what you can do; you won't be able to just change your 'mindset' when the little voice is talking to you . . . What is funny about pressing on is that it is innately human: When you are learning how to walk, you don't all of a sudden decide it is too hard and quit. Even though we are born entirely helpless, we have the instinct to move forward in the face of adversity."[19]

---

16   Personal correspondence, February 15, 2018.

17   *New York Daily News*, January 29, 2009.

18   Personal correspondence, June 19, 2018.

19   Interview, October 15, 2018.

Needless to say, exactly what makes a person resilient is a subject of debate. The Marine Corps calls it "endurance," and lists it as one of its fourteen leadership traits. The idea is the same: the ability to overcome mind-boggling challenges like pain, fatigue, stress, and hardship. Others in the military prefer to call it "hardiness." Retired army colonel and former West Point lecturer Paul T. Bartone described a hardy person as someone who has "a strong sense of life and work commitment, a greater belief of control, and more openness to change and challenges in life."[20]

Not only are resilient people open to change—they actually welcome it. This is why elite fighting units consider creative thinking essential. According to Dick Couch, author of *Chosen Soldier: The Making of a Special Forces Warrior*, "The Special Forces are looking for more than someone who is tough and smart and plays well with others. They are looking for adaptability and flexibility, men who can look at a given task and come up with any number of ways to solve it."

When speaking of hardiness, Paul Bartone stressed the importance of a feeling of control. And Lt. Col. Dave Grossman, a public speaker and co-author of *Assassination Generation*, actually called it an "internal locus of control," which is an idea that harks back to Julian Rotter, a professor of psychology at the University of Connecticut. Rotter's idea states that certain individuals feel they are in control of their own fate for the most part. "You identify the things you can control and do them," Grossman says. "Identify the things you can't control and let go of them." Using the breath gives us practical application of this "letting go." Steven Southwick, professor of psychiatry at the Yale School of Medicine and author of the book *Resilience: The Science of Mastering Life's Greatest Challenges*, tells us how to manage stressful situations by acquiring "the ability to observe your thoughts and emotions without necessarily becoming them . . . Your brain can run you ragged with your thoughts and one of the tricks to managing stress is to recognize that you don't have to respond to every single one. You choose what you want to focus on."

---

20 "Personality Hardiness as a Predictor of Officer Cadet Leadership Performance," November 1999, RTO MP-55. http://www.dtic.mil.

EXPERT ADVICE

Top sports psychologists like Jonathan Fader, author of *Life as Sport: What Top Athletes Can Teach You About How to Win in Life,* and Nate Zinsser, director of the Performance Psychology Program at West Point, both include the importance of breath in their presentations. This discernment gives you control over yourself, the only thing you can control in a chaotic and unpredictable environment such as combat. Without this control you can go into shock, go ballistic and lose your aim, your mission, or even your life. Controlling your arousal level is essential to survival. And you can control your arousal with your breathing. Lt. Col. Dave Grossman, includes breathing as the mechanism that keeps your frontal lobe from being hijacked during high stress. (An apt analogy is his saying that "When it does, it's like yelling at your puppy through a mail slot.") His simple recommendation is to pause and take a sip of water.

DO THIS NOW

Why does taking a sip of water calm you down? You have to stop breathing for a second or two in order to swallow. This pause takes a critical few seconds as your tongue levers to help you swallow and forces you to stop what you were about to do to rev your nervous system—to hyperventilate. The water forces you to pause, and this critical second interrupts the cycle of panic and allows you to take back the steering wheel.

"Pilot etiquette" is the practice and steadfast rule that regardless of the circumstance you speak clearly and calmly, explains retired Chief of Staff of the Chicago Police Department James Roussell. Roussell has thirty-nine years of service in the infantry and intelligence sector of the USMC and has specialized in gang tactical units. The control of speech makes for more efficient communication, but underneath it is control of the exhale, making for a practice that encourages calm even in chaos. Knowledge of your breath, then, is the best tool you have to connect with your internal control system, align your attitude with your goals, and keep your arousal where you want it given the situation.

AROUSAL CONTROL

"Resilience is the ability to return to normalcy," according to Jen Baker, Director of Athletics and Recreation at John Hopkins University, a graduate of the U.S. Naval Academy. "It's . . . your ability to bounce back and thrive, replace worry with objective things, to navigate and take next steps forward.[21] It's not that you can't mourn," she adds, because "disappointment is an affirmation that you are invested." Baker uses her military background and knowledge of yoga and the breath to cultivate personal and team resilience.[22]

RESILIENCE: IS IT IN YOU?

Good news: you don't have to be born with it. You can build it. Psychologist and resilience expert Ann Masten in *American Psychologist* describes resilience as "ordinary magic" because it's something that can be developed with practice and intent.

KEEPING THE BUTTERFLIES IN FORMATION

As Al Lee and Don Campbell so astutely point out in their book *Perfect Breathing,* "For performing artists, the breath not only governs the quality of the physical performance, but it also plays a key role in managing the accompanying fear, anxiety, excitement, and adrenaline— keeping the butterflies flying in formation as it were—so that they can be used to unleash the muse and fuel the creativity and spontaneity of the performance."

ACTIVE MEDITATION IS A RESILIENCY TOOL

Being tough means being able to tolerate discomfort and be effective; resilient means being able to bounce back from it. Integrating an active breathing meditation into your regimen gives you both. Anything that challenges you to be stronger is going to make you stronger, both physically and emotionally. And success begets success. Resilience is different because it's also about how fast you *recover*. It sounds like something you own or don't, but the fact is you can add a practical active recovery to your day, meaning your immune system will be boosted and keep you healthier when others are sick. It means you *truly* recover from a hard day (not just buckle up

---

21   Interview, December 10, 2018.

22   From a presentation on Friday, March 29, 2019, at the LUF Summit, Annapolis, Maryland.

and seem as if you do); it means you work out hard one day and are able to "refresh" in order to do it again tomorrow.

INJURY

At some point something is going to break, and it will feel as if your body betrayed you. But the law of attraction does not apply when it comes to injuries, and thinking and planning for them will not make them more likely to happen.

POINTS TO KEEP IN MIND:

1. Develop your intuition by integrating breathing and active meditation into your practice. You'll be more likely to hear the difference when your prefrontal cortex tells you to put the weight down and pause, or when your reptilian brain, jacked on pre-workout juice, is screaming along with Rage Against the Machine and taunting you and luring you into a danger zone.
2. The day after you get injured, grab your crutches and head over to the gym first thing in the morning. If you hurt your knee, blast your chest and back. If you hurt your shoulder, plan for a month of legs. You are at high risk for depression if exercising has been your go-to, so the last thing you should do is hit the snooze button and sulk.
3. Do the harder breathing exercises until you sweat through your T-shirt. Every day. Bellows Breath, Exhale Pulsations, balloons, O2 trainer, meditation. Your body and brain are probably pissed and fermenting in anger and stagnant lymph—and the best way to get rid of it and not lose your conditioning is to work the ten pounds of muscle that are your breathing muscles.
4. And finally, sign up for some volunteer work and get some perspective. No one wants to hang out with an irritable, injured baby. The world is full of cancer and injustice; your torn meniscus or strained rotator cuff will heal (or not) but the world will keep turning.

"Old rib cage fractures, bruises and strains often lead to an apical (shallow, vertical) breath . . . then comes disuse of the diaphragm and fibrosis or scar tissue along the intercostal muscles which lead to dysfunctional breathing."

—John Zapanta, PT, DPT,
Colorado in Motion

Pain is a complex process that involves nerve receptors, neurology, the central nervous system, and—yes—breathing. The sensation of pain can have a profound effect on one's breathing patterns and vice versa. Al Lee and Don Campbell in *Perfect Breathing* report that, "People in pain will often take multiple short, fast inhales with a long exhale." But on the flip side, slow breathing has repeatedly shown itself to be an effective pain reducer. It's not entirely clear why this happens; researchers just regularly observe that it does. A German study that appeared in *Pain Medicine* in 2012 indicates that relaxation might be part of the reason. Researchers saw that when subjects performed deep, slow breathing techniques, their pain threshold went up. Consequently, whatever the underlying mechanism may be, deep breathing is recommended as a treatment for chronic pain and back pain and for people recovering from surgery.[23]

"The car accident crushed my leg, and all I could think about was if I'd get to play basketball again. If I hadn't had breathing exercises to do I know I would have lost my mind. The thoughts that I was falling behind, that I'd lose my conditioning, that I was helpless "waiting to heal," were making me depressed, irritable, and anxious. I learned to do a whole breathing workout from my hospital bed. I would sweat, soak the sheets, but I'd get the same intensity and endorphins of a workout. Once I was able to start rehab and swim, my conditioning was not terrible and I'd managed to keep myself from getting really depressed."

—Tony S.

---

23   Ohayon, Maurice M. and Julia Sting. "Prevalence and comorbidity of chronic pain in the German general population." *Pain Medicine*, April 2012.

ITS: INTERRUPTING THE STRESS

Distressed people breathe erratically, unbalancing both their biochemical selves and further putting themselves in a dominant sympathetic state. Unfortunately, this is a self-reinforcing circular pattern, one that may have started with a stressful event or with bad breathing styles, modes, and patterns. Figuring out the why is less important than stopping the loop of stress/anxiety and auxiliary muscle's dominant erratic breathing. Interrupt the stress (or better yet, stop it as you see it rising) by breathing low and wide.

Dan McGuire is a UK-based stuttering expert, who seeks to interrupt the stress when working with his patients. McGuire theorizes that the crural diaphragm is chronically contracting in response to fear in those who stutter, causing great distress: "You can spend years desensitizing fear or work on using the diaphragm."[24]

Remember: mantras only "talk" to your brain (you are trying to convince yourself of something); you aren't calming yourself if your heart rate is still elevated. The other danger is if the mantras don't ring true and they actually feed into an "imposter syndrome" (similar to the mantra in golf that you are having fun or the one in finance—that it's just chips).

PUBLIC SPEAKING IS A SPORT

Balance and Energize	Breathe like an *Opera Singer*	Avoid the *"Cheerleader Syndrome"*	*Audible* Exhale

As you review your breathing mechanics and strength, put some thought into the basics of public speaking[25] as a sport, summarized by the acronym BOCA.

1. ***Balance and Energize.*** A biomechanically sound breath means

24   For more details on the McGuire Program, check out his book *Beyond Stuttering.*

25   Heather Lyle, author of *Vocal Yoga*, is a little gold mine of information about breathing for speaking.

feeling more balanced and better energy. A power pose will get you to the mic but the lower breath will keep you calm.

2. *Breathe like an Opera Singer.* Once you have really mastered a 360-degree breath, you'll be able to breathe laterally and through your back like a rock star. Check out opera singer Maria Callas for someone to look up to.

3. *Avoid the "Cheerleader Syndrome."* If you are a teacher and are taking a narrow Vertical Breath while straining to motivate your class, over time you can damage your vocal cords. Better breathing means better projecting and modulating.

4. *Audible Exhale.* The most important takeaway? Your vocalizations are auditory exhales. If public speaking makes you anxious, then this is probably a good part of the problem. A more efficient inhale will give you the exhale that will allow you to make it to the end of the sentence gracefully.

FREQUENTLY ASKED QUESTIONS

Q: **When I panic, I start to hyperventilate and I realize I breathe through my mouth. Any advice?**

A: *Patrick McKeown is your go-to for everything related to overbreathing. He is an expert in Buteyko Breathing, and is a big proponent of Nasal Breathing.*

NOTE FOR THE COACH

There's no app for pain: Younger generations of athletes are more at risk for injuries because they are so externally driven. Stakes are higher; and the inner voice that helps one pull back when it's the sort of pain that is information (not pain needed for optimization) is barely audible to them.

There is a moment when you waver about being hopeful that you're healing. Whereas we've found, once "healed," the fear of re-injury comes looming. The sadness and frustration might worsen to a clinical depression that warrants treatment. Such as when the preperformance jitters manifest as full-out panic attacks; when your genetics and life experience collide and you find yourself

self-medicating. Your mental health is part of your game; make sure you put time and effort into it as well.

FROM FIELD TO STAGE

Statistics show that if you are an athlete, you probably will end up in some kind of situation, sports or otherwise, that puts you in front of a group, or a camera, or into a leadership position. And leaders have to speak, make speeches, motivate, and rule over kingdoms and corporations, large and small. So, whether you go pro and need to speak at charity events, you end up coaching and needing to inspire your athletes, or if you go corporate as an entrepreneur of some sort, your talent of being strong and fast now has to switch to eloquent.

> Two German researchers, Aleksandra Ćwiek and Petra Wagner, found that there are two types of breathing pauses, non-breathing pauses and turn-taking cues.[26]

SPEAKERS SPEAK OUT

Steve Uria, founder of Switch Playground:

> *"If you told me I was going to go from a military drill sergeant to leading an exercise class with one hundred people and pumping music I'd have told you you were crazy. I went from a drill sergeant to a motivational speaker. And while you think they have a lot in common, fact is that everything I knew about how to convey a message had to be ripped down and built up again. My tone, humor, nuance, connectivity. None of those things mattered when I had a platoon in front of me. I had to find examples that would resonate with the audience, be likable, sound intelligent, and care what the reaction was. I wasn't giving direction anymore."[27]*

26   Cwiek, A., and Wagner, P. "Investigating the communicative function of breathing and non-breathing 'silent' pauses." Conference paper, 2016.

27   Personal communication, April 27, 2019.

Marcus Kowal, professional mixed martial arts athlete and author of *Life Is a Moment*:

> *"I've never been shy, but now the topic I was talking about was intensely personal. My infant son's death at the hands of a drunk driver got national attention. I was mourning, trying to support my wife and keep moving. Forming a nonprofit to help change drunk driving laws meant I was both fueled by my anger and sadness, but also had to manage getting a clear message to the public while juggling intense emotions."*[28]

Jason Ferruggia, author and strength and conditioning expert:

> *"If you would have told my meathead self twenty years ago that I'd actually enjoy standing in front of a group, motivating them and making them laugh with information on how to be their best selves I'd have thought you were high. I was shy, angry, and liked training solo with loud music in my ears. Twenty years later I am at the polar opposite of the spectrum. I relish quality interaction. Before I thought I had to be a lone wolf to be effective.*[29]

Don Saladino, celebrity trainer and fitness expert:

> *"I like being under the pressure of live TV. In videos you could do second and third takes. When it's live and interactive there you have to negotiate personalities— juggle a lot of different expectations and intangibles like how you are carrying yourself . . . I quickly learned that this challenge fueled me."*[30]

---

28   Interview, January 8, 2019. My first book on breathing was dedicated to Marcus's nonprofit, Liam's Life, whose mission is both to stop drunk driving and support organ donation.

29   Interview, February 4, 2019.

30   Interview, March 18, 2019.

ARE YOU REVVING?

Watch a group of people talking. You'll notice how one person spends their time almost holding their breathing and constantly "revving."

DO THIS NOW

Read along with a great speech, using the same intonations as an exercise. Hearing your own voice through your ears is often distracting and anxiety provoking. Make sure you get used to hearing your voice out loud so that it doesn't distract you.

And do your homework. Maybe you've decided to sign up for an improv class because you heard it's a good skill for speaking, or you are prepping to speak at a wedding. Kymberlee Weil, a speaking strategist at Strategic Samurai, points out, "When we feel nervous or anxious or fearful, we often hold our breath or breathe very shallow and this can exacerbate our anxiety."

BIBLIOGRAPHY

Ancell, Henry. *A Treatise on Tuberculosis: The Constitutional Origin of Consumption and Scrofula*. Forgotten Books, 2018.

Anderson, Robert H. et al. "Cardiac anatomy revisited." *Journal of Anatomy* 205 (no. 3) (2004):159–77.

Aschwanden, Christie. *What the Athlete in All of Us Can Learn from the Strange Science of Recovery*. W. W. Norton & Company, 2019.

Bækkerud, F. H., F. Solberg, and I. M. Leinan. "Comparison of Three Popular Exercise Modalities on V̇O2max in Overweight and Obese." *Medicine & Science in Sports & Exercise* 48, no. 3 (2016):491–98.

Baker, A. B. "Artificial Respiration, the History of an Idea." *Medical History* 15, no. 4 (1971):331–51.

Bassett, David R. "Scientific Contributions of A. V. Hill: Exercise Physiology Pioneer." *Journal of Applied Physiology* 93, no. 5 (2002):1567–82.

Benton, Marc L., and Neil S. Friedman. "Treatment of obstructive sleep apnea syndrome with nasal positive airway pressure improves golf performance." *Journal of Clinical Sleep Medicine*, 9 (2013):1237–42.

Bompa, Tudor and Carlo Buzzichelli. *Periodization Training for Sports*. Human Kinetics, 2015.

Borkowski, S., J. C. Bernardo, and G. K. Hung. "Effect of Psychological Pressure on Eye, Head, Heart & Breathing Responses During the Golf Putting Stroke." *Journal of Behavioral Optometry* 20, no 2 (2009):37–41.

Bowman, Katy. *Diastasis Recti: The Whole Body Solution to Abdominal Weakness and Separation*. Propriometrics Press, 2016.

Boyd, Jenna et al. "Mindfulness-Based Treatments for Post-Traumatic Stress Disorder: A Review of the Treatment Literature and Neurobiological Evidence." *Journal of Psychiatry & Neuroscience* 42, no. 1 (2017):7–25.

Bradley, H., and J. Esformes. "Breathing Pattern Disorders and

Functional Movement." *Journal of Sports Physical Therapy* 9, no. 1 (2014):28–39.

Bramble, D. M., and D. E. Lieberman. "Endurance running and the evolution of Homo." *Nature* 432 (2004):345–52.

Chaline, Eric. *The Temple of Perfection: A History of the Gym*. Reaktion Books Ltd., 2015.

Cholewicki, J., et al. "Intra-Abdominal Pressure Mechanism for Stabilizing the Lumbar Spine." *Journal of Biomechanics* 32, no. 1 (1999):13–17.

Coast, J. R., and C. C. Cline. "The effect of chest wall restriction on exercise capacity." *Respirology*, 9 (2004):197–203.

Coates, Budd with Claire Kowalchik. *Running on Air: The Revolutionary Way to Run Better by Breathing Smarter*. Rodale Inc., 2013.

Coleman, Loren. *Suicide Clusters*. Faber & Faber, 1987.

Couch, Dick. *Chosen Soldier: The Making of a Special Forces Warrior*. Three Rivers Press, 2008.

Cressey, Eric. *Maximum Strength*. Da Capo Lifelong Books, 2008.

Cuddy, Amy. *Presence: Bringing Your Boldest Self to Your Biggest Challenges*. Little, Brown and Company, 2015.

Cwiek, A., and P. Wagner. "Investigating the communicative function of breathing and non-breathing 'silent' pauses." Conference paper, 2016.

Dempsey, J., et al. "Consequences of Exercise-Induced Respiratory Muscle Work." *Respiratory Physiology & Neurobiology* 151, no. 2–3 (2006):242–50.

Divine, Mark. *Unbeatable Mind*. Create Space Independent Publishing Platform, 2015.

———. *The Way of the SEAL*. Reader's Digest, 2018.

Dooley, Kathy. *An Inner Journey*. Create Space Independent Publishing Platform, 2016.

Draper, N., et al. "Effects of Active Recovery on Lactate Concentration, Heart Rate and RPE in Climbing." *Journal of Sports Science & Medicine* 5 (2006):97–105.

European Lung Foundation. "Your lungs and exercise." *Breathe* 12, no. 1 (2016):97–100.

Evans, Janet. *Total Swimming*. Human Genetics, 2007.

Fader, Jonathan. *Life as Sport: What Top Athletes Can Teach You About How to Win in Life.* Da Capo Lifelong Books, 2016.

Falsone, Sue. *Bridging the Gap from Rehab to Performance.* On Target Publishers, 2018.

Farhi, Donna. *The Breathing Book.* Holt Paperbacks, 1996.

Ferruggia, Jason. *Fit to Fight.* Avery, 2008.

Finn, C. "Rehabilitation of Low Back Pain in Golfers: From Diagnosis to Return to Sport." *Sports Health* 5, no. 4 (2013):313–19.

Frank, C., et al. "Dynamic Neuromuscular Stabilization & Sports Rehabilitation." *International Journal of Sports Physical Therapy* 8 (2013):62–73.

Froning, Rich. *First: What It Takes to Win.* Tyndall House Publishers, 2013.

Gaines, Thomas. *Vitalic Breathing.* Kissinger Publishing, 2003.

Galpin, Andy. *Unplugged: Evolve from Technology to Upgrade Your Fitness, Performance and Consciousness.* Victory Belt Publishing, 2017.

Glick, J. C., and Alice Atalanta. *Meditations of an Army Ranger: A Warrior Philosophy for Everyone.* Lightning Press, 2019.

Goosey-Tolfrey, V., E. Foden, and C. Perret. "Effects of Inspiratory Muscle Training on Respiratory Function and Repetitive Sprint Performance in Wheelchair Basketball Players." *British Journal of Sports Medicine* 44 (2010):665–68.

Gothe, Neha P., et al. "The Effects of an 8-week Hatha Yoga Intervention on Executive Function in Older Adults." *Journals of Gerontology* 69, no. 9 (2014):1109–16.

Graham, Deborah, and Jon Stabler. *The 8 Traits of Champion Golfers: How to Develop the Mental Game of a Pro.* Simon & Schuster, 1999.

Grossman, David. *On Killing: The Psychological Cost of Learning to Kill in War and Society.* Back Bay Books, 2009.

———. *Assassination Generation.* Little, Brown and Company, 2016.

Haj Ghanbari, B., et al. "Effects of respiratory muscle training on performance in athletes: a systematic review with meta-analyses." *Journal of Strength and Conditioning Research* 27, no. 6 (2013):1643–63.

Hidden, N. R., W. H. Finch, D. Leib, and E. L. Dugan. "Effects of Fatigue on Golf Performance." *Sports Biomechanics* 11, no. 2 (2012):190–96.

Hildebrandt, L. K., et al. "Cognitive Flexibility, Heart Rate Variability, and Resilience Predict Fine-grained Regulation of Arousal During Prolonged Threat." *Psychophysiology* (2016):880–90.

Hill, E. E., et al. "Exercise and circulating cortisol levels: The intensity threshold effect." *Journal of Endocrinological Investigation* 31, 7 (2008):587–91.

Hyson, Sean. *The Men's Health Encyclopedia of Muscle*. Rodale, 2018.

Ikuo, Homma and Yuri Masaoka. "Breathing rhythms and emotions." *Experimental Physiology*, 2008.

Jensen, K., S. Jørgensen, and L. Johansen. "A metabolic cart for measurement of oxygen uptake during human exercise using inspiratory flow rate." *European Journal of Applied Physiology*, vol. 87 (2002):202–14.

Jerath, R., et al. "Physiology of Long Pranayamic Breathing: Neural Respiratory Elements May Provide a Mechanism That Explains How Slow Deep Breathing Shifts the Autonomic Nervous System." *Medical Hypotheses* 67, no. 3 (2006):566–71.

John, Don. *Now What: The Ongoing Pursuit of Improved Performance*. On Target Publications, 2017.

Junger, Sebastian. *Tribe*. Twelve, 2016.

Kapus, J., A. Usaj, and M. Lomax. "Adaptation of endurance training with a reduced breathing frequency." *Journal of Sports Science & Medicine* 12, no. 4 (2013):744–52.

Kardian, Steve. *New Superpower for Women*. Touchstone, 2017.

Kenney, Bradford. *Shaking Medicine*. Destiny Books, 2007.

Kilding, A. E., S. Brown, and A. K. McConnell. "Inspiratory Muscle Training Improves 100 and 200 m Swimming Performance." *European Journal of Applied Physiology* 108 (2010):505–11.

Klentrou, P., J. Slack, and B. Roy. "Effects of Exercise Training with Weighted Vests on Bone Turnover and Isokinetic Strength in Postmenopausal Women." *Journal of Aging and Physical Activity* 15 (2007):287–99.

Kufahl, Pamela. "IHRSA Reports 57 Million Health Club Members, $27.6 Billion in Industry Revenue in 2016." *Club Industry*, April 14, 2017, p. 4.

Lee, Al, and Don Campbell. *Perfect Breathing: Transform Your Life One Breath at a Time*. Sterling Publishing, 2009.

Lee, Diane. *The Pelvic Girdle*. Churchill Livingston, 2010.

Liebenberg, L. "Persistence Hunting by Modern Hunter Gatherers." *Current Anthropology* 47, no. 6 (2006):1017–26.

Lieberman, Philip and Robert McCarthy. "Tracking the Evolution of Language and Speech." *Expedition Magazine (Penn Museum)* 49, no. 2 (2007):15–20.

Lin, H. C., C. S. Chou, and T. C. Hsu. "Stress Fractures of the Ribs in Amateur Golf Players." *Zhonghua Yi Xue Za Zhi* 54, no. 1 (1994):33–37.

Lloyd, Robin. "Gasping for Air." *Scientific American* 316 (2017):26–27.

Lomax, M. "Inspiratory muscle training, altitude and arterial oxygen desaturation: A preliminary investigation." *Aviation Space, and Environmental Medicine*, 81, no. 5 (2010):498–501.

Lopes, Felipe A. S., et al. "The effect of active recovery on power performance during the bench press exercise." *Journal of Human Kinetics* 40 (2014):161–69.

Lyle, Heather. *Vocal Yoga*. Blue Cat Music and Publishing, 2010.

Macklem, P. T., R. G. Fraser, and W. G. Brown. "Bronchial Pressure Measurements in Emphysema and Bronchitis." *Journal of Clinical Investigations* 44 (1965):897–905.

MacLean, Katherine A., et al. "Intensive Meditation Training Improves Perceptual Discrimination and Sustained Attention." *Psychological Science* 21, no. 6 (2010):829–39.

Masten, Ann S. "Ordinary magic: Resilience processes in development." *American Psychologist* 56, no. 3 (2001):227–38.

McConnell, Alison. *Breathe Strong, Perform Better*. Human Kinetics, 2011.

———. *Respiratory Muscle Training: Theory and Practice*. Churchill Livingston, 2013.

McDermott, W. J. et al. "Running training and adaptive strategies of locomotor-respiratory coordination." *European Journal of Applied Physiology* 89 (2003):435–45.

McGill, Stuart M. *Low Back Disorders*. Human Kinetics, 2015.

———. *Ultimate Back Fitness and Performance*. Stuart McGill, 2004.

McGlashan, Lara. "Amelia Boone: The Queen of Pain." *Muscle & Performance*. September 26, 2017.

McGuire, David. *Beyond Stammering*. Souvenir Press Ltd., 2003.

Melnychuk, C. M., et al. "Coupling of Respiration and Attention via the Locus Coeruleus: Effects of Meditation and Pranayama." *Psychophysiology* 55 (2018):124–33.

Michaelson, Joana, et al. "Effects of Two Different Recovery Postures During High-Intensity Interval Training." *Journal of the American College of Sports Medicine* 4, no. 4 (2019): 23–27.

Mika, Anna. "Comparison of Recovery Strategies on Muscle Performance After Fatiguing Exercise." *American Journal of Physical Medicine & Rehabilitation* 86, no. 6 (2007):474–81.

Monplaisir, Marc. *The Complete Rowing Machine Workout Program*. Front Runners Publications, 2014.

Mumford P. W., A. C. Tribby, and C. N. Poole. "Effect of Caffeine on Golf Performance and Fatigue During a Competitive Tournament." *Medicine & Science in Sports & Exercise* 48, no. 1 (2016):132–38.

Myers, Thomas W. *Anatomy Trains: Myofascial Meridians for Manual and Movement Therapists*. Churchill Livingston, 2014.

Neumann, D., et al. "The relationship between skill level and patterns in cardiac and respiratory activity during golf putting." *International Journal of Psychophysiology* 72 (2019):276–82.

Noakes, Tim. "Fatigue Is a Brain-Derived Emotion That Regulates the Exercise Behavior to Ensure the Protection of Whole Body Homeostasis." *Frontiers in Physiology* 3, no. 82 (2012):216–38.

Ogden, C., et al. "Mean Body Weight, Height, and Body Mass Index, United States 1960–2002." *ADV Data* 347, no. 1 (2004):1–17.

Ohayona, M. M. and J. Sting. "Prevalence and comorbidity of chronic pain in the German general population." *Journal of Psychiatric Research* 45, no. 4 (2012):444–50.

Pacenski, Tony. *A Story of Invisible Power*. Create Space Independent Publishing Platform, 2016.

Paulson, Erik, et al. *Rough and Tumble: The History of American Submission*. Blue Plate Books, 2010.

Peper, Erik. "Biofeedback, breathing and health." Biofeedback Federation of Europe, November 2017.

Peper, E. et al. "Which quiets the mind more quickly and increases HRV: Toning or mindfulness?" *NeuroRegulation*, 6, no. 3 (2019):128–33.

——— et al. "The Physiological Correlates of Body Piercing by a Yoga Master: Control of Pain and Bleeding." *Subtle Energies & Energy Medicine Journal* 14, no. 3 (2005):223–37.

Philippen, P. B. and B. H. Lobinger. "Understanding the Yips in Golf: Thoughts, Feelings, and Focus of Attention in Yips-Affected Golfers." *The Sport Psychologist* 26 (2012):325–40.

Potkin, R., et al. "Effects of glossopharyngeal insufflation on cardiac function." *Journal of Applied Physiology* 103, no. 3 (2007):823–27.

Puthoff, M. L., B. J. Darter, D. H. Nielsen. "The Effect of Weighted Vest Walking on Metabolic Responses and Ground Reaction Forces." *Journal of Medicine & Science in Sports & Exercise* 38, no. 4 (2006):746–52.

Reyes, Rudy. *Hero Living: Seven Strides to Awaken Your Infinite Power*. Celebra, 2010.

Riccio, Lucius. *Golf's Pace of Play Bible*. Three/45 Golf Association, 2013.

Rippetoe, Mark. *Starting Strength: Basic Barbell Training*. The Aasgaard Company, 2007.

Rogers, April J., et al. "Obstructive Sleep Apnea Among Players in the National Football League: A Scoping Review." *Journal of Sleep Disorders & Therapy* 6, no. 5 (2017):278–82.

Romer, L. M., A. K. McConnell, and D. A. Jones. "Effects of Inspiratory Muscle Training on Time-Trial Performance in Trained Cyclists." *Journal of Sports Sciences* 20, no. 7 (2002):547–90.

———. "Specificity and Reversibility of Inspiratory Muscle Training." *Medicine & Science in Sports & Exercise* 35, no. 2 (2003): 237–44.

Rooks, J. D., et al. "We Are Talking About Practice: The Influence of Mindfulness vs. Relaxation Training on Athletes' Attention and Well-Being over High-Demand Intervals." *Journal of Cognitive Enhancement* 1 (2017):1–41.

Sandow, Eugen. *Life Is Movement*. Create Space Independent Publishing Platform, 2012.

Sarno, John. *The Mindbody Prescription*. Warner Books, 1999.

Schmidt, Norman B., et al. "Exploring Human Freeze Responses to a Threat Stressor." *Journal of Behavior Therapy and Experimental Psychiatry* 39, no. 3 (2007):292–304.

Sharma, G., and J. Goodwin. "Effect of Aging on Respiratory System Physiology and Immunology." *Clinical Interventions in Aging* 1, no. 3 (2006):253–60.

Sheel, A. W., P. A. Derchak, and D. F. Pegelow. "Threshold effects of respiratory muscle work on limb vascular resistance." *American Journal of Physiology-Heart and Circulatory Physiology* 282 (2002):1732–38.

Sheridan, Sam. *A Fighter's Heart: One Man's Journey Through the World of Fighting*. Grove Press, 2008.

Smith, Stew. *The Complete Guide to Navy SEAL Fitness*. Hatherleigh Press, 2008.

Southwick, Steven. *Resilience: The Science of Mastering Life's Greatest Challenges*. Cambridge University Press, 2012.

Superrich, B., H. Fricke, and M. Marées. "Does respiratory muscle training increase physical performance?" *Military Medicine* 174, no. 9 (2009):977–82.

Starrett, Kelly. *On Becoming a Supple Leopard*. Victory Belt Publishing, 2015.

Streeter, Chris, et al. "Effects of Yoga on Thalamic Gamma-Aminobutyric Acid, Mood and Depression: Analysis of Two Randomized Controlled Trials." *Neuropsychiatry* 8, no. 6 (2018): 1923–28.

Thomson, A. "The Role of Negative Pressure Ventilation." *Archives of Disease in Childhood* 77 (1997):545–58.

Tong, T. K., and P. K. Chung. "The Effect of Inspiratory Muscle Training on High-Intensity, Intermittent Running Performance to Exhaustion." *Applied Physiology, Nutrition, and Metabolism* 33 (2008):671–81.

Tsai, Jang-Zern, et al. "Left-Right Asymmetry in Spectral Characteristics of Lung Sounds Detected Using a Dual-Channel Auscultation System in Healthy Young Adults." *Sensors* 17, no. 6 (2017):13–23.

Tsatsouline, Pavel. *Kettlebell Simple & Sinister*. StrongFirst, Inc., 2013.

———. *The Naked Warrior*. Dragon Door Publications, 2003.

Tyagi, A., and M. Cohen. "Yoga and Heart Rate Variability: A Comprehensive Review of the Literature." *International Journal of Yoga* 9, no. 2 (2016):97–113.

Valcheva, Zornitsa, et al. "The role of mouth breathing on dentition development and formation." *The Journal of IMAG* 24, no. 1 (2018):1878–82.

Vasiliev, Vladimir, with Scott Meredith. *Let Every Breath . . . Secrets of the Russian Breath Masters*. Russian Martial Art, 2006.

Verges, S., P. Fiore, and G. Nantermoz. "Respiratory Muscle Training in Athletes with Spinal Cord Injury." *International Journal of Sports Medicine* (2009):193–212.

Verstegen, Mark, with Pete Williams. *Core Performance: The Revolutionary Workout Program to Transform Your Body*. Rodale, 2004.

Vickers, Joan. "Neuroscience of the Quiet Eye in Golf Putting." *International Journal of Golf Science* 1 (2012):2–9.

Vincent, Lynn, and Sara Vladic. *Indianapolis: The True Story of the Worst Sea Disaster in U.S. Naval History and the Fifty-Year Fight to Exonerate an Innocent Man*. Simon & Schuster, 2018.

Volker, Busch, et al. "The Effect of Deep and Slow Breathing on Pain Perception, Autonomic Activity, and Mood Processing—An Experimental Study," *Pain Medicine* 13, no. 2, (2012):215–228.

Walker, William (aka Yogi Ramacharaka). *Hatha Yoga*. Cornerstone Publishers, 2015.

Weitzberg, E., and Jon O. N. Lundberg. "Humming Greatly Increases Nasal Nitric Oxide." *American Journal of Respiratory and Critical Care Medicine* 166 (2002):144–45.

West, J. B., R. R. Watson, and Z. Fu. "The Human Lung: Did

Evolution Get It Wrong?" *European Respiratory Journal* 29 (January 2007):11–17.

Wilmer, Henry H. B., et al. "Smartphones and Cognition: A Review of Research Exploring the Links Between Mobile Technology Habits and Cognitive Functioning." *Frontiers in Psychology*, 8 (2017):1–16.

Illustration Captions with Text from *The Anatomy of Breathing* by Blandine Calais

Figure 3.1, p. 26: The diaphragm is a large muscular and fibrous wall which simultaneously separates and connects the thorax and the abdomen. The diaphragm is sometimes compared to a parachute, an upside-down bowl, a shower cap, or a jellyfish.

Figure 3.2, p. 27: Anatomy of the diaphragm. The diaphragm has a fibrous center part, which is called the central tendon, around which are muscular fibers arranged in a beam-like fashion. These fibers attach to the entire circumference of the rib cage. Transversus abdominis: partner of the diaphragm. This is the muscle that helps you "narrow your waist." This action is greatest at the level of the costoiliac region where its fibers are the biggest. It is not good for the muscle to be the dominant participant here, because it exerts a strong pressure on the lower part of the abdomen. That is why it is often necessary to coordinate its action with other abdominal muscles.

Figure 3.3, p. 29: Rectus abdominis: the only abdominal muscle that does not pull apart the linea alba. It participates in anterior costal expiration by dropping the sternum. It participates in intensive expirations by raising the pubic bone (an action used sometimes for totally closing the anterior abdomen). It completes the rectus sheath of the large abdominal muscles. The advantage of using the rectus abdominis is that it pulls without pulling the abdomen apart, as do the large abdominal muscles. This is a good example to use when "sucking in the stomach" during expiration (think of doing this action "from the front"). The rectus abdominis always participates at the beginning of each exhalation by using its lowest fibers (in conjunction with those of the other abdominal muscles) to hold and suck in the lowest, most anterior portion of the abdomen.

Figure 5.1, p. 50: The first contractile action of the intercostals is to bring the intercostal spaces closer together and to make the ribs slightly glide on each other.

Figure 6.2, p. 60: Abdominal muscles. The muscles support and surround the abdomen. There are four of them on the left and on the right: The rectus abdominal in the front. Three layers of large muscles that lay on top of each other on the sides.

Figure 7.1, p. 72: The lumbar vertebrae extend from the pelvis upward and form the posterior wall of the abdominal cavity. They connect the pelvis to the thoracic cage.

The five lumbar vertebrae are massive, and many respiratory muscles attach to them: the diaphragm, transverse abdominus, quadratus lumborum, and serratus posterior inferior.

Because the pelvis and thoracic cage are linked together through the lumbar vertebrae, they behave independently. The movement of either one will influence the contents—the organs—of the other, shaping them and also influencing the breathing.

Figure 7.2, p. 75: The pelvis is a bony structure at the base of the trunk, which looks both like a container for the organs and also like a solid ring which connects the trunk with the lower limbs. It consists of four bones: the two hip bones, the sacrum, and the coccyx.

Figure 7.3, p. 78: The deep layer of the pelvic muscles. These muscles are located deeper and above the preceding layer, situated in the lesser pelvis, and closer to the internal organs . . . and form a hammock, holding all the pelvic organs within their concave surface. They respond passively (elastic) and actively (tonic) to variations in abdominal pressure.

Figure 11.1, p. 124: Rectus abdominis. Among other actions, the rectus abdominis participates in expiration in the following ways: it participates in anterior costal expiration by dropping the sternum. It participates in intensive expirations by raising the pubic bone (an action used sometimes for totally closing the anterior abdomen). This is a good muscle to use when "sucking in the stomach" during expiration (think of doing this action "from the front").

Figure 12.1, p. 137: Spine. The spine serves as a solid support structure: for the neck and the head, where the inspiratory muscles attach: the sternocleidomastoid (SCM), the scalenes, and the serratus posterior superior. For the rib cage, which is connected to the spine through about forty articulations and numerous muscles; the rib cage can move around the spine or remain immobilized. For the lumbar region, which contains the abdominal organs that are impacted by the diaphragm and the abdominal muscles. For the sacrum, the back region of the pelvis where the muscles of the pelvic floor attach.

INDEX